God's Will Be Done
Volume III

Moral Healing Through the Most Beautiful Names:
The Practice of Spiritual Chivalry

Laleh Bakhtiar

The Institute of Traditional
Psychoethics and Guidance

Book Designer
Liaquat Ali

Library of Congress Cataloging in Publication Data

Bakhtiar, Laleh
Moral Healing Through the Most Beautiful Names

Includes bibliographical references.
1. Psychology, Religious. 2. Consciousness.
3. Theology. 4. Ethics. I. Bakhtiar, Laleh. II. Title
BL53.U45 200'.19 75.16302
ISBN: 1-871031-40-0

Published by
THE INSTITUTE OF TRADITIONAL
PSYCHOETHICS AND GUIDANCE
CHICAGO, IL

Distributed by
KAZI PUBLICATIONS, INC., (USA)
3023 W. BELMONT AVENUE
CHICAGO IL 60618
TEL: (312) 267-7001; FAX: (312) 267-7002

Contents

Preface VII
Overview XIII
Part I: Nourishment of Spiritual Warriors: Knowledge of God Through Theoethics 1

Part II: The Process of Moral Healing for Spiritual Warriors Through Psychoethics 65
Chapter One: Moral Healing of the Attraction to Pleasure Function of the Self Through Acquiring Temperance 67
Stage 1: Resolve, Submission 71
Stage 2: Hope-Fear 72
Stage 3: Piety 74
Stage 4: Moderation 75
Stage 5: Tranquillity 76
Stage 6: Spiritual Poverty/Altruism 77
Stage 7: Self-Restraint 78
Chapter Two: Moral Healing of the Avoidance of Harm/Pain Function of the Self Through Acquiring Courage 79
Stage 1: Compassion 83
Stage 2: Moral Reasonableness 85
Stage 3: Thankfulness 87
Stage 4: Vigilance 89
Stage 5: Trust 90
Stage 6: Repentance 91
Stage 7: Patience 93
Chapter 3: Moral Healing of the Cognitive Function of Self Through Acquiring Wisdom 95
Stage 1: Aspiration 99
Stage 2: Self-Examination 101
Stage 3: Truthfulness 103
Stage 4: Contentment 105
Stage 5: Unity/Constancy 106
Stage 6: Sincerity 107
Stage 7: Remembrance 108
Chapter 4: Centering the Self with Justice 111

Part III: The Actions of Spiritual Warriors: Proof of Moral Healing Through Socioethics 113

Chapter One: Social Awakening by Emptying the Self of Everything But the Desire to Grow Closer to God 119

Chapter Two: Entering the Creative Process 131

Chapter Three: Counseling to the Positive and Trying to Prevent the Development of the Negative 137

Chapter Four: Developing the Moral Reasonableness of a Religiously Cultured Monotheist 149

Chapter Five: Using Their Spiritual Power to Help Others 159

Chapter Six: God's Trustee 171

Chapter Seven: Perfecting Their Instinctive Perception Through Noble Character Development 183

Chapter Eight: Perfecting Their Instinctive Motivation Through Their Actions 193

Chapter Nine: Moving Towards Servanthood by Serving God's Creation 207

Chapter Ten: Serving as a Guide and Teacher to Others 217

Conclusion 227

Appendices:

A: List of the Order of the 99 Most Beautiful Names, Translation, Transliteration, Quality and Number Symbolism (West and East) 235

B. List of the Translation of the 99 Most Beautiful Names, The Order, Division and Summary Description of Role in Theoethics, Psychoethics and Socioethics 238

C. List of the Number Symbolism (East) of the 99 Most Beautiful Names, Translation, Transliteration, Quality, Number Symbolism (West), Division and Elemental Properties 249

D. List of the Quality of the 99 Most Beautiful Names, Translation, Transliteration, Number Symbolism (West and East), Divisions and Elemental Properties 252 and Elements

E. List of the Translation of the 99 Most Beautiful Names, Their Letters and Number Symbolism (East), and Their Elemental Properties 255

F. List of the Translation of the 99 Most Beautiful Names, Their Letters and Number Symbolism (West) and Their Elemental Properties 258

G. List of the Transliteration of the 99 Most Beautiful Names and Their Invocation (dhikr) with an Index to Special Properties 261

Notes 271

Bibliography 275

Index 277

To my beloveds
—Saied and Samira—
whom I pray
–with the Will of God—
continue to receive
God's Blessings, Guidance and Grace

PREFACE

The key to morally healing the self for the spiritual warrior[1] is through actualizing the Most Beautiful Names, following the Signs, "*To God belong the Names Most Beautiful so call on Him*[2] *by them*" (7:179) and "*To Him belong the Names Most Beautiful*" (20:7). This, in turn, purifies the heart, the center of consciousness so that the Light of the original nature can be made manifest. Through the presence of this Light, the heart follows reason and turns itself towards the spiritual instead of following the passions and turning towards the material world. If spiritual warriors manifest or express these Names and Qualities in their interactions with others, they are called noble character traits and in relation to the self, they are referred to as praiseworthy character traits. Spiritual warriors come to learn that their mercy should precede their wrath; too much justice (*'adl*) without mercy (*raḥama*) will result in tyranny; being too compassionate (*raḥīm*) without justice (*'adl*) will result in moral disorder. Everything, then, including their relationship with self and others has to be in balance, at the mean, kept in moderation.

The practices of spiritual warriors are many but they all relate in one way or another to the Most Beautiful Names of God. The Most Beautiful Names—traditionally Ninety-Nine in number although infinite in Reality—serve as the "*Signs upon the horizons and within themselves*" (41:53) which they read in order to gain knowledge of them; to thereby undertake a process whereby they are able to assume a portion of them; and, finally, to manifest them in their actions in relationship to God's creatures—animate and inanimate.

Knowledge of the Most Beautiful Names may be attained in a multiple of ways—formal and informal. It matters not to the spiritual warrior how he or she gains this knowledge, but, rather, the emphasis is upon the necessity to learn. It may be through formal schooling, learning as many of the Divine Names and Qualities as possible and a future career in theology. It may be through a teacher, a master, who explains the Real workings of the universe to the spiritual warrior a few at a time. Still, it may be through self-taught knowledge learned through reading or learned through an intuitive understanding of the workings of Reality. It is to attain knowledge of the Name or Quality in its Absolute sense in order to put the relative, negative idol/ego in its place in relation to the Absolute (theoethics).

Part I: Nourishment of Spiritual Warriors: Knowledge of God Through Theoethics presents one method of gaining knowledge of the Most Beautiful Names. It is a translation of the part of Algazel's *Maqṣad al-asnā fī sharḥ asmā' Allāh al-ḥusnā* which relates directly to the Ninety-Nine Most Beautiful Names as they appear in a well-known reliable Tradition (*ḥadith*).

There are many traditional divisions of the Most Beautiful Names practiced by the various Sufi orders—Names of Beauty, Names of Majesty, Names of Perfection and so forth. The divisions which serve to further moral healing is one found in the Traditions (*aḥadith*) of the Messenger in which he describes the Names and Qualities by which God Self-discloses to Self, to creation and to humanity.

Moral healing through theoethics is effected by the realization that only God has these Names and Qualities in the absolute sense allowing spiritual warriors to sense real "servantness" and "creatureliness" in relation to God. When people consider their "self" without considering the Divine Source, they manifest their false self or ego which is the satanic aspect of self. Moral healing takes place through theoethics when spiritual warriors "see things as they really are" and realize their place in the vast universe is that of trustee and not absolute power.

This serves as nourishment for the spiritual warrior who then tries, through moral healing of the self, to assume a portion of the Ninety-Nine Most Beautiful

Names (psychoethics). Spiritual warriors do this as a moral obligation which is twofold. First of all, the moral obligation to morally heal arises from the covenant which the human being accepted when God blew His Spirit within and secondly in order to fulfill the conditions to be an effective trustee of nature in which God is the Trust-Giver.

Part II: The Process of Moral Healing for Spiritual Warriors Through Psychoethics presents the same Ninety-Nine Most Beautiful Names but with an emphasis on the healing process of assuming the Names. Those Names and Qualities through which God Self-discloses to creation are ones through which spiritual warriors learn temperance or, in religious rather than philosophical terms, altruism or giving to others what one oneself needs (*ithār*) which is one of the highest virtues or positive traits of spiritual chivalry. Those Names and Qualities through which God Self-discloses to humanity are ones through which spiritual warriors learn courage or trust in God. Finally, those Names and Qualities through which God Self-discloses to Self are ones through which spiritual warriors learn wisdom or the belief in the One God.

Temperance—altruism— in the view of spiritual chivalry arises from the circle of self when the instinctive attraction to pleasure or preservation of the species is disciplined by reason to moderation. Courage—trust in God—arises when the instinctive avoidance of harm/pain or preservation of the individual is disciplined by reason to moderation. Wisdom—belief in the One God—arises from the circle of self in the view of spiritual chivalry when the instinctive ability to reason is disciplined and oriented to the preservation of the eternal possibility of self.

Part III: The Actions of Spiritual Warriors: Proof of Moral Healing Through Socioethics presents the same Ninety-Nine Most Beautiful Names as the other two parts, but here the Presence of a Name in spiritual warriors' relations to others is proof of having morally healed. It is to be found in their actions forming the basis for a socioethics that has the potential to heal society as a whole when each individual follows it. The stories used to further express each name in its social aspect are translated from Jalal al-Din Rūmī's *Mathnawī* and *Fīhī MāFī* ("In It Is What Is In It") unless otherwise indicated.

The basic practice of spiritual chivalry that runs through all three aspects of assuming a portion of the Most Beautiful Names—knowledge, process, actions—is that of *dhikr* or remembrance of God, in particular, in its relationship to the traditional sciences of letters and numbers.

A word should be mentioned about the graphics which appear throughout this work. Moral healing through the Most Beautiful Names is a traditional practice connected to what the Sufis call *wajh Allāh* (the Presence or Face of God),[3] known as the Enneagram in the West. Volume I of *God's Will Be Done: Traditional Psychoethics and Personality Paradigm* develops the monotheistic theory of personality which is expressed in the Sign of the Presence of God. Volume II of *God's Will Be Done: Moral Healer's Handbook: The Psychology of Spiritual Chivalry* develops the traditional theory of counseling. This, in the monotheistic perspective, is to heal morally again expressed through the Sign of the Presence of God. Not only is this Sign an image of the self within but it is manifested in the universe in the coordinations of Saturn and Jupiter in relation to the Zodiac which is first presented to the West by the author in Volume II of this trilogy.

Volume III of *God's Will Be Done: Moral Healing Through the Most Beautiful Names: The Practice of Spiritual Chivalry*, the present work, again ties in with the image of the Sign of the Presence of God.

Part I: The Nourishment of Spiritual Warriors: Knowledge of God Through Theoethics shows the Arabic equivalent of each Divine Name or Quality which is focused on in "remembering" or "reciting" that Name or Quality in terms of Self-disclosure to creation, to humanity or in Self; the numerical significance of the Name or Quality is based on the science of numbers which differed in the East and in the West of the Islamic world; and the elemental property of a Name or Quality based on the science of letters (hot, cold, wet or dry).

The graphics of Part II: The Process of Moral Healing of Spiritual Warriors Through Psychoethics show what part of the self is being healed according to the diagram of the Sign of the Presence of God and each Name or Quality as it appears in the Tradition of the Ninety-Nine Most Beautiful Names.

Part III: The Actions of Spiritual Warriors: Proof of Moral Healing Through Socioethics indicates the division of the Name or Quality in the Sign of the Presence of God through the graphics of wisdom (Names Self-disclosed to Self), temperance (Names Self-disclosed to creation) and courage (Names Self-disclosed to humanity).

There is a final intention to the text and graphics of this work and that is to give a sense of Divine infiniteness in terms of multiplicity of manifestation while holding to an underlying sense of unity, centeredness, balance and harmony. No matter how spiritual warriors relate to the Most Beautiful Names, the possibilities inherent in being able to assume a portion of them are overwhelming and awe-inspiring.

Spiritual warriors then traditionally use the experiential knowledge gained through knowledge-process-action to transform whatever material they have at hand into so many works of sacred art—whether it be the self or a material at hand which they as members of a craft guild produce. They may also be members of a neighborhood watch group in which case they protect their neighborhoods as moral keepers of the peace or they may be members of a traditional athletic association in which case their sense of moral goodness is used in their competitions with other athletes. They have traditionally also manifested as knights and members of various Sufi orders where service to others is emphasized.

*****

I wish to acknowledge the help of my children: Mani, Davar and Susan, Karim, Shervin and Faroukh for their continued moral support along with that of my brother, Jamshid Bakhtiar and sister, Shireen Bakhtiar (pen name, White Cloud); to the readers of this work: Jamshid Bakhtiar, Christian Fitzpatrick, Riazuddin Riaz, Ali John Comegys and Muhammad al-Akili for their valuable comments and criticisms; to my teachers: Javad Nurbakhsh, Seyyed Hossein Nasr and Jamshid Bakhtiar; and to KAZI Publications for the continued encouragement board members have given me.

Overview

Traditional Ethics

The science of ethics is considered to be the most basic requirement before attempting to learn or practice any other science because all sciences are dependent upon ethics.

Naraqi, an exponent of psychoethics, writes,

> In fact, in the past, philosophers did not consider any of the other fields of learning to be truly independent sciences. They believed that without the science of psychoethics, mastery over any other science is not only devoid of any value, but it would, in fact, lead to the obstruction of insight and ultimate destruction of those who pursue it. That is why it has been said knowledge is the thickest of veils which prevents the human being seeing the real nature of things.[1]

Nasir al-Din Tusi, another scholar of ethics, says,

> The subject matter of this science, then, is the human 'self' in as much as from it can proceed, according to its free-will, acts fair and praiseworthy or negative and destructive. This being so, it must be known what the self is, where its perfection lies, what the functions are by which, if used in moderation, it attains what it seeks, namely perfection of nature [in its method of operation or God's Will] and what prevents it from reaching that perfection. In other words, one needs to know how to purify the [heart] and avoid seducing it, thereby bringing about its prosperity rather than its failure....[2]

The Relative Self

In the view of spiritual chivalry, the self differs from the body and is considered to be independent of it. It is created (not pre-eternal as Plato and Aristotle held). It can only be known, understood, and studied indirectly with the cognitive power of reason or mental perception, observing the activities that originate from it. It manifests itself in states which are constantly changing and need to be centered in order to be able to perfect its nature. Its function is to perceive intelligibles by its own essence and to regulate and control the physical body by means of faculties and organs. It is not a body nor is it physical nor is it sensed by any of the senses. It includes the vegetative soul (nutritive faculty, augmentative faculty, and faculty of generation and corruption), animal soul (faculty of perception and motivation), and human soul which, in turn, contains four major aspects: the spirit (*rūh*), the heart (*qalb*), the intellect (*'aql*), and the passions or irrational aspects of self.

The spirit which is contained within the heart is subject to neither amount, quantity, nor measure. The spirit receives life or Grace which is distributed to the heart in the form of the Most Beautiful Names. Grace from the spirit manifested in the heart through the Most Beautiful Names give life, knowledge, and cognitive abilities to the heart so that the heart can become conscious of grace.

The heart, then, is the seat of consciousness of God and is capable of progressing the self towards perfection. It is called *qalb* meaning "turning, revolving, inverting" because it contains two worlds within itself—the physical and the spiritual and constantly turns from one to the other. Through the process of psychoethics, the self is healed when consciousness of God within the self succeeds in turning the heart constantly towards the spiritual and away from the material.

The material aspect of self is called the passions or irrational functions. They are held in common between human beings and animals. In both cases, the passions arise out of motivational impulses. Motivational impulses manifest in the passions rule animals to the extent that they completely submit to nature in its method of operation. They have no choice.

When, however, the heart had been gifted by the

Divine Spirit with consciousness, it also received two requirements of consciousness: conscience and free-will. While the consciousness of the heart is the highest stage of cognition, conscience is the highest stage of perception and free-will, that of motivational impulses. With the appearance of free-will, the self, unlike animals, becomes free to choose to submit to nature in its method of operation or not, choose to become conscious of God or not. When reason is habituated and disciplined to receive impulses from the imagination and deliberate with free-will and conscience instead of the imagination by passing reason and going directly to the passions, reason rules the self. Otherwise, the passions rule.

THE PROCESS OF MORAL HEALING

Moral healing through the Most Beautiful Names is to effect this process. That is, once spiritual warriors gain knowledge of the meaning of 'self' (psychoethics), the purpose behind their creation, and they gain knowledge of God's Self-disclosure through the Most Beautiful Names (theoethics), they realize that they did not create their 'self' nor any other person nor the universe. That is, there must be a Creator and if the Creator were not one, there would be disagreement in its governance which is not the case. The one Creator created the world in balance and harmony. The trust of nature and maintaining its balance and harmony was entrusted to the human being who is the only creature to have received the infusion of the divine Spirit or consciousness of God.

ACCEPTING THE COVENANT

It is only the human being who was asked to form the covenant with God, which it did. This is expressed in the verse, "*And when your Lord took the seed of the children of Adam from their loins,*" and asked, "'*Am I not your Lord?*'" and the human being answered, "'*Yea. We do bear witness*'" (7:173).

ACCEPTING THE TRUST

Having accepted the covenant, God breathed the Spirit within and the human being became the trustee (*wakil*) of nature: "*We offered the trust to the heavens and the earth and the mountains, but they refused to carry it and were afraid of it, and the human being carried it*" (33:72). Accepting the trust then set up a moral responsibility to carry out the trust on the part of the human being. In return for morally healing the self to meet the requirements of a trustee and then carrying out the duties of the trust, the self receives salvation and eternal life. This trusteeship includes three relationships: between the human self and God's Self-disclosure (theoethics); between the human self and human self (psychoethics); and between self and all of nature including other human beings (socioethics).

BALANCING THE NATURAL DISPOSITION BY DISCIPLINING THE FALSE SELF OR EGO DEVELOPED THROUGH THE NURTURING PROCESS

The human being enters the world with a nature originated by God (*fiṭrat Allāh*). This natural disposition is instinctively programmed to be a balanced trustee. Being balanced means choosing through their will to perfect nature in its mode of operation or God's Will by purifying the heart so that it can become conscious of "things as they really are" in order to preserve the equilibrium. Perfect balance is based in the norms of monotheism—where it says, for instance, "*...weigh things with the balance...*"—and actualized by God's Messenger as an example of a perfected human being.

Following the model of creation, moral healing occurs according to spiritual chivalry, when the self is in a state of balance or equilibrium. This balance is a relative mean, the furthest point between two extremes. If a person lives in moderation, in balance and preserves the self in a positive state, he or she will, at the end, depart completely from the body. The result will be freedom from suffering and attaining the joy of the beauty of eternal salvation.

Moral balance is traditionally defined as, "The intermediate state in all things which is to be praised but they must incline sometimes towards the excess, sometimes towards the deficiency for so shall they most easily hit balance and what is right."[3]

According to Algazel, this is not impossible to attain based on the Quranic verse, "*There is not one of you but shall pass through it [the fire]. That is a fixed ordinance of the Lord. Then We shall rescue those who kept from [the negative] and leave the [negatively disposed] crouching there.*".

It is the nurturing process which turns spiritual warriors away from their natural disposition of balanced trustee by appealing to their material aspect of self or natural passions instead of their spiritual aspect of self or natural reasoning powers. The passions, referred to in the Quran as *nafs ammārah* , are attraction to pleasure (affect, preserve the species) and avoidance of pain (behavior, preserve the individual).

Attraction to pleasure is the most basic instinct within the human being and is unconscious, in the greatest need of discipline because its nature is greedy and often aggressive in the pursuit of its desires and wishes. When it is not controlled by reason, it produces inappropriate desires and lust, inappropriate in the sense of being beyond God's bounds, being beyond 'the common good'. Avoidance of harm/pain is considered to be preconscious and capable of being trained. It is defensive—preserve the individual from harm/pain—manifested in anger. When it is not controlled by reason, it produces inappropriate anger and tends towards conquest, killing and violence.

These two forces of the passions make up the material aspect of the human being. As they are part of the material world, they are formed out of a combination of the basic properties of cold, hot, dry, and humid which are contained in pairs in the elements earth, fire, water, and air. Each of these elements contain two basic properties in pairs. Earth is by nature cold and dry; water is cold and humid; air is hot and humid; and fire is hot and dry.

Attraction to pleasure is a downward inclination and tendency and therefore its nature is similar to that of earth and water—cold dry/humid. Avoidance of harm/pain or anger (self-exaltation and arrogance) is an upward movement and tendency and therefore similar in nature to air and fire—hot and dry/humid. As the nature of heat dries up moisture, only the properties of cold or hot are taken into consideration. These two functions—attraction to pleasure which is cold by nature and avoidance of harm/pain which is hot by nature—are both necessary for sustaining of life but they have to be maintained in a state of balance.

From this it can be seen that the most sensitive area of the healing process is training the self to seek deliberation with reason which in turn calls upon free-will and conscience for counsel. This is when the self is healed, giving birth to consciousness of God in the heart. When the self is not so trained or when free-will and conscience are contacted without the input of reason, the passions or attraction to pleasure or avoidance of harm/pain rule through the idol/ego—the satanic aspect of self. This is when negative traits appear which are imbalanced in the self in terms of either quantity or quality. When the imbalance is in terms of quantity, it can either be an excess or a deficiency. When the imbalance is in terms of quality, the self falls outside the circle of unity and needs to return to it before even attempting moral healing. In terms of cognition, this is considered to be unconsciousness (not knowing that you do not know); in terms of attraction to pleasure it is to manifest envy and in terms of avoidance of harm/pain it is to have fear of other than God.

Negative traits of the attraction to pleasure function in terms of quantity—excess or deficiency—include traits manifesting inappropriate desires and wishes like coveting the world and wealth, affluence and opulence, avarice, greed, treachery, debauchery, and lying. Negative traits of the avoidance of harm/pain function include inappropriate anger, lack of endurance and self-depreciation, timidity, lack of a sense of dignity, hastiness, self-conceit and vanity, revengefulness, violence, ill-temperedness, enmity and hostility, arrogance, boastfulness, rebelliousness, fanaticism, and injustice. Negative traits of reason which develop when it is not trained to regulate the self include simple ignorance of Reality resulting in multitheism, compound ignorance of Reality resulting in disbelief, perplexity and doubt, deceit and trickery resulting in a state of hypocrisy.[4]

Moral healing begins when the spiritual warrior returns to the nature originated by God. The return is seen as a struggle, the greater struggle with the self. On one side is reason and the other, the passions, which are struggling for the attention of the heart. In order to return to the nature originated by God, the spiritual warrior first needs to know self.

KNOWLEDGE OF THE RELATIVE SELF LEADS TO KNOWLEDGE OF GOD

According to Algazel, there are three ways to obtain self-knowledge. The first is to share in the knowledge of the meanings of God's Most Beautiful Names as Signs upon the horizon and within the self through witnessing and unveiling. Through **knowledge** gained in this way, the essential reality of the Name is understood by spiritual warriors. When they look within themselves, they become certain about some qualities that they may contain which they recognize as God's manifestation of Self-disclosure. Faith gained in this way is far deeper and more meaningful than faith adopted from one's parents or teachers through imitation (*taqlīd*).

Second, to so honor and respect these qualities that spiritual warriors long to possess them in order to grow closer to the Real, the Truth (al-Ḥaqq) in terms of quality, not place. This longing draws spiritual warriors into a **process** whereby the self becomes receptive to assume a portion of the Most Beautiful Names. If the heart is filled with respect for a quality and enlightened and illuminated because of this respect, it necessarily follows that spiritual warriors develop a longing for the quality. Out of this longing, a passionate love develops for that perfection. Spiritual warriors then seek to assimilate that quality to the extent possible.

Two obstacles may prevent this: first inadequate information and knowledge of certainty that the quality is one of perfection and secondly, if the heart is filled with love for something else—like their own ego or worldly attachments. Moral healing begins, then, by emptying their heart of desiring anything but God in order to be able to contemplate God's perfect qualities. The self must be freed from inappropriate anger and desires which are the animal qualities within the human form. The seed of longing, which is knowledge, is then planted. If the heart is not empty of the passions, the seed will not bear fruit.

Third, with the goal being to draw closer to God, spiritual warriors. emptied of all desires but for God, relate to society through **action** which is the basis for a socioethics that brings further moral healing among others. Imitating the Divinity to the extent humanly possible, the actions of spiritual warriors are proof of them having morally healed and thereby attaining the rank of trustee of nature and self.

Healing Techniques Through the Most Beautiful Names

Healing techniques through the Most Beautiful Names as so many methods of preparing the self to receive Grace begin with certain preparations and then include techniques like remembrance or invocation of the Names based on the sciences of letters and numbers.

Preparation

In addition to the necessity for ablution and the recommendation for major ablution, spiritual warriors who wish to morally heal the self and purify the heart are recommend not to eat meat on the day of God's remembrance (*dhikr*). They should choose a clean place for which they also have permission to use. It is best to be alone, at night, from midnight to the dawn prayer. With eyes closed, there should be no interruptions during the remembrance. Those who take no liquids after six pm on the day of remembrance are more likely to have real dreams.

It is recommended to begin by reciting "*la illaha illa lah muhammadan rasullah*" ("there is no god but God, Muhammad is the Messenger of God") 700 times. Once the seeker is ready to recite one of God's Names, they call to that name with the ejaculation "*yā*" (oh) to appeal to It.

REMEMBRANCE OR INVOCATION

Remembrance of the Most Beautiful Names is to understand the name, picture it in its calligraphic, Arabic form, judge it, reflect on it, hold it in memory and recite it often.[5] The seeker begins with the remembrance of the Most Beautiful Names through the tongue. Effort is exerted to place the remembrance in the heart. Little by little the recitation proceeds without effort as the seeker moves away from the movement of the tongue into seeing the word as if the word were engulfing the person. The seeker at this point is still conscious of the experience as a receptive subject, in a state of consciousness of the name being recited or invoked.

Spiritual warriors have been told by God to remember God often in the morning and evening."*Remember Me (God) and I will remember you,*" (2:152) and "*Those who believe in their hearts being at rest in God's remembrance—in God's remembrance are at rest the hearts of those who believe and do righteous deeds; theirs is a blessedness and a fair resort*" (13:28).

There are ten stages to follow in prayer according to

Algazel:[6]

1. Choosing the best time such as the two festivals—one at the end of the month of fasting (Ramadan) and one the day of sacrifice at the end of the pilgrimage to Makkah—or Friday[7] or the time of daybreak.

2. After the prescribed prayers. Traditions emphasizing this are: "Verily the prescribed prayer is offered during the best hours so you should remember after the prescribed prayers."[8] "Remembrance made between the call to the prescribed prayer and the moment of standing in prescribed prayer is never rejected."[9] "The human being is nearest to God when he prostrates so make many supplications at that time"[10] And, "Verily I refrained from reciting the Quran while bowing and prostrating. While you are bowing, glorify the Lord. While you are prostrating, make supplication earnestly for it is a suitable time for your request to be heard."[11]

3. Pray to the direction of the prescribed prayers (*qiblah*) with hands held so high that the whiteness of the armpits can be seen. Algazel quotes the Tradition, "Verily your Lord is living and generous; He feels too ashamed when His servants raise their hands toward Him to return them empty"[12] and "When the Messenger stretched his hands in supplication, he never withdrew them until he wiped his face with them."[13]

4. The voice should be modulated between silent and loud. This is confirmed by the verse, "*Call on Him humbly and secretly*" (7:55).

5. There should be no attempt to show off to another person. Maintaining balance is important even in prayer as a Tradition states, "There will come people who go beyond the proper bounds in remembrance and prescribed purification."[14]

6. Approach with humbleness, submissiveness, longing, and fear. This is confirmed by the verse, "*They were competing with one another in doing good deeds and calling unto Us in longing and in fear*" (21:90).

7. Be direct and unconditional sincerely believing you

will receive a response. Traditions are many which confirm this including, "Let not any of you in prayer say, 'Oh God forgive me if You will! Have mercy on me if You will!'. Instead, ask directly because there is no one who compels Him."[15] "When any of you supplicates, let him make big requests for nothing competes with God in greatness."[16] "Supplicate to God with firm conviction of His response. Know that God never answers the supplication of him whose heart is heedless."[17]

8. Supplicate earnestly and repeat your request three times. When the Messenger supplicated, he supplicated three times and when he asked, he asked three times.[18] One should not wait impatiently for the response, "Any of you will be answered so long as he is not so anxious as to complain saying, 'I have prayed but I have not been answered yet.' So when you supplicate, ask God for much because you are supplicating to a Generous One."[19]

9. Begin with the invocation of God not with the prayer. The Messenger never began supplication without this invocation, "Glory be to my Lord, the Highest, the Most Exalted, the Bestower (*subhan Allāhi rabbi al-'alī al-a'la al-wahhāb*)."[20]

10. Inward attitude should be one of repentance, rejection of negative traits and turning toward God with the utmost effort.

According to the Traditions, if spiritual warriors know a specific area where they need healing, they recite that name frequently or a prescribed number of times anytime or at a specific time.[21]

THE SCIENCE OF LETTERS

The science of letters gives a quality to each of the twenty-eight letters of the Arabic alphabet based on basic properties of nature of hot, cold, wet and dry. In healing the body, they serve as the basis for determining what foods need to be eaten in order to preserve the physical self in balance. If the body has fallen out of balance and been moved by a hot illness, for instance, the healer will recommend cold foods to counterbalance the illness or a lesser degree of food by its nature found to be hot or cold. These properties underlie moral healing, as well, through invoking the Most Beautiful Names according to their natural property based on their letters.

The letters of fire (hot and dry) are:
alif, h, ṭ, m, f, s and *dh*

The letters of air (hot and humid) are:
b, w, y, n, ḍ, t and *ẓ*

The letters of water (cold and humid) are:
j, z, k, ṣ, q, th , and *gh*.

The letters of earth (cold and dry) are:
d, ḥ, l, 'ayn, r, kh and *sh*.

The letters are broken down (*taksīr*) according to the natural property in the Name. Some of the Names are in balance while others are cold or hot. Dry/humid are not considered because heat dries.[22]

The science of letters (*simīyā* meaning signs) is also considered as a sacred science by the spiritual warrior because it is based on a sacred language—Arabic—through which God chose to reveal the Quran. While nature is seen as the "cosmogonic Quran" (*takwīnī*), the "recorded Quran" (*tadwīnī*) is composed of letters and sounds. As Ibn al-'Arabī says,

> The Universe is a vast book; the characters of this book are all written, in principle, with the same ink and transcribed on the eternal Table by the Divine Pen; all are transcribed simultaneously and inseparably; for that reason the essential phenomena hidden in the 'Secret of the Secrets' were given the name of 'transcendent letters'. And these transcendent letters, that is to say, all creatures, after having been virtually condensed in the Divine Omniscience, were carried down on the Divine Breath to the lower lines and composed and formed the manifested Universe.[23]

The inner relationship between the science of numbers and the science of letters has been expressed by al-Būnī:

> Numbers symbolize the spiritual world and letters symbolize the corporeal world...Know that the secrets of God and the objects of His Science, the subtle and the gross realities, the reality of on-high and of the here-below, and those of the angelic world are of two kinds, numbers and letters. The secrets of the letters are in the numbers and the theophanies of the numbers are in the letters. Numbers are the realities of on-high due to spiritual entities and letters belong to the circles of material and angelic realities. Numbers are the secret of works and letters the secret of actions.[24]

The numbers 1-9 [25] on the Sign of the Presence of God are symbols of the Arabic alphabet. The alphabet corresponds to the same four elements and their four qualities as do the planets, the universe seen as unfolding through the sounds of the letters. While all of creation is the emanation from 1, each number, while more basic than the elements and their qualities, are seen as repeats of unity.

Ibn Khaldun explains:

> The Sufis wrote systematic works on Sufism and Sufi terminology. They believed in the gradual descent of existence from the One. They believed that verbal perfection consists in helping the spirits of the spheres and the stars (through words). The natures and secrets of the letters are alive in the words, while the words, in turn, are correspondingly alive in the created things. The created things have been moving in the different stages of creation and telling its secrets since the first creation. These Sufi beliefs caused the science of the secrets of the letters to originate...Al-Būnī, Ibn al-'Arabī and others in their wake wrote numerous works on it. These authors assume that the result and fruit of letter magic is that the Divine souls are active in the world of nature by means of the Beautiful Names of God and the

Divine expressions that originate from the letters comprising the secrets that are alive in the created things.

The authorities on letters then differed as to the secret of the activity lying in the letters. Some of them assumed that it was due to inherent temper. They divided the letters into four groups corresponding to the elements. Each element had its own group of letters. Through this group of letters it can be active actively and passively. A technical procedure, which they call breaking down (*taksīr*) classifies the letters as the elements are classified, as fiery, airy, watery and earthy. The *alif* is fiery, *b* airy, *j* watery and *d* earthy. Then it starts again with the next letter and so on through the whole alphabet and the sequence of the elements.... The fiery letters serve to repel cold diseases and to increase the power of heat whatever desired, either in the sensual (physical) or in the astrological sense. Thus, for instance, one may want to increase the power of Mars for warfare, the killing of enemies and aggressiveness.

In the same way, the watery letters serve to repel hot diseases, such as fevers and others, and to increase the cold powers, wherever desired, either in the sensual (physical) sense or in the astrological sense. Thus, for instance, one may want to increase the power of the moon and so on.

Others assumed that the secret of the activity that lies in the letters was their numerical proportion. The letters of the alphabet indicate numerical values which by convention and nature are generally accepted to be inherent in them. Thus, there exists a relationship between the letters mentioned and *d, m,* and *t*. The latter group of letters indicates four and the proportion of four to two is that of two to one. Then, there are magic squares for words as there are for numbers. Each group of letters has a particular kind of magic square which fits it in the view either of the numerical value of the figure or of the numerical value of the letters. Activity based on letters thus merges with that based on numbers because there exists a relationship between letters and numbers.

The real significance of the relationship existing between letters and natural humors and between letters and numbers is difficult to understand. It is not a matter of science or reasoning. According to the authorities, it is based on mystical experience and the removal of the veil. Al-Būnī says, 'One should not think that one can get at the secret of the letters with the help of logical reasoning. One gets to it with the help of vision and Divine aid.'

The fact that it is possible to be active in the world of nature with the help of the letters and the words composed of them and that the created things can be influenced in this way, cannot be denied. It is confirmed by continuous tradition on the authority of man...

The activity of people who work with words is the effect of the Divine Light and the support of the Lord which they obtain through struggle and the removal of the veil. Thus, nature is forced to work for them and does so willingly with no attempt at disobedience. Their activity needs no support from the spherical powers or anything else, because the support it has is of a higher order than all that.... People who work with words use the most extensive exercise possible. It is not for the purpose of being active in the existing things since that is a veil standing between them and their real task. Such activity comes to them accidentally as an act of Divine Grace. A person who works with words may have no knowledge of the secrets of God and the realities of divinity which is the result of vision and the removal of the veil. He may restrict himself to the various relationships between words and the natures of letters and expressions and he may become active with them in this capacity....

Many people wanted to obtain the ability to be active in a way that would have nothing to do with any involvement in disbelief (*kufr*) and the practice of it. They turned their exercise into one that was legal according to the Law. It consisted of exercises of remembrance (*dhikr*) exercises and prayers from the Quran and the Hadith. They learned which of these

> things were appropriate for their particular need from the aforementioned division of the world with its essences, attributes and actions according to the influences of the seven planets. In addition, they also selected the days and hours appropriate to the distribution of the influence of the planets...They kept to a legal kind of devotion because of its general and honest character.[26]

THE SCIENCE OF NUMBERS

Just as the twenty-eight letters of the Arabic alphabet have healing powers through their properties, they also have numerical power based on the verse, *"We send down not a thing but its number is known"* (15:21).

The numbers assigned to each letter differ in the East and the West for six of the letters.[27] The two systems are:

West						East					
alif	1	y	10	q	100	alif	1	y	10	q	100
b	2	k	20	r	200	b	2	k	20	r	200
j	3	l	30	s	300	j	3	l	30	sh	300
d	4	m	40	t	400	d	4	m	40	t	400
h	5	n	50	th	500	h	5	n	50	th	500
w	6	ṣ	60	kh	600	w	6	s	60	kh	600
z	7	ayn	70	dh	700	z	7	ayn	70	dh	700
ḥ	8	f	80	ẓ	800	ḥ	8	f	80	ḍ	800
ṭ	9	ḍ	90	gh	900	ṭ	9	ṣ	90	ẓ	900
	sh 1000						gh 1000				

Each of the Most Beautiful Names has, in this way, an inherent number so that if healing is sought through the science of numbers, a correspondence is sought with that of the Most Beautiful Names. This method allows for a correspondence between the Most Beautiful Names that do not appear in the specific form in the Quran with the other Names that do appear in the Quran. The Name is broken down into hundreds, tens, and units and then the letter equivalent is found which is used to effect physical or moral healing.

Part I: Nourishment of Spiritual Warriors: Knowledge of God Through Theoethics

"We shall show them Our Signs
upon the horizons and within themselves
until it is clear to them
that it is the Real (the Truth)" (41:53).

God Self-disclosed through the manifestation of the Most Beautiful Names of which one Tradition relates the following Ninety-Nine Names of **Allāh**:

(1) The Merciful (al-Raḥmān)
(2) The Compassionate (al-Raḥīm)
(3) The Sovereign (al-Malik)
(4) The Holy (al-Quddūs)
(5) The Flawless (al-Salām)
(6) The Giver of Faith (al-Mu'min)
(7) The Guardian (al-Muhaymin)
(8) The Incomparable (al-'Azīz)
(9) The Compeller (al-Jabbār)
(10) The Proud (al-Mutakabbir)
(11) The Creator (al-Khāliq),
(12) The Maker of Perfect Harmony (al-Bāri'),
(13) The Shaper of Unique Beauty (al-Muṣawwir)
(14) The Forgiver (al-Ghaffār)
(15) The Subduer (al-Qahhār)
(16) The Bestower (al-Wahhāb)
(17) The Provider (al-Razzāq)
(18) The Opener (al-Fattāḥ)
(19) The Knower (al-'Alīm)
(20) The Constrictor (al-Qābiḍ)
(21) The Expander (al-Bāsiṭ)
(22) The Abaser (al-Khāfiḍ)
(23) The Exalter (al-Rāfi')
(24) The Honorer (al-Mu'izz),
(25) The Dishonerer (Mudhill)
(26) The All-Hearing (al-Samī')
(27) The All-Seeing (al-Baṣīr)
(28) The Arbiter (al-Ḥakam)
(29) The Just (al-'Adl)
(30) The Subtle (al-Laṭīf)
(31) The Aware (al-Khabīr)
(32) The Forebearing (al-Ḥalīm)
(33) The Magnificent (al-'Aẓīm)
(34) The Concealer of Faults (al-Ghafūr)
(35) The Rewarder of Thankfulness (al-Shakūr)

(36) The Highest (al-'Alī)
(37) The Great (al-Kabīr)
(38) The Preserver (al-Ḥāfiẓ)
(39) The Maintainer (al-Muqīt)
(40) The Reckoner (al-Ḥasīb)
(41) The Majestic (al-Jalīl)
(42) The Generous (al-Karīm)
(43) The Vigilant (al-Raqīb)
(44) The Responder to Prayer (al-Mujīb);
(45) The Vast (al-Wāsi')
(46) The Wise (al-Ḥakīm)
(47) The Loving (al-Wadūd)
(48) The Glorious (al-Majīd)
(49) The Resurrector (al-Bā'ith)
(50) The Witness (al-Shahīd)
(51) The Truth (al-Ḥaqq)
(52) The Trustee (al-Wakīl)
(53) The Strong (al-Qawī)
(54) The Firm (al-Matīn)
(55) The Friend (al-Walī)
(56) The Praised (al-Ḥamīd)
(57) The Appraiser (al-Muḥṣī)
(58) The Beginner (al-Mubdi')
(59) The Restorer (al-Mu'īd);
(60) The Giver of Life (Muḥyī)
(61) The Slayer (Mumīt)
(62) The Living (al-Ḥayy)
(63) The Self-Existing (al-Qayyūm)
(64) The Resourceful (al-Wājid)
(65) The Noble (al-Mājid)
(66) The Unique (al-Wāḥid)
(67) The One (al-Aḥad)
(68) The Eternal (al-Ṣamad)
(69) The Able (al-Qādīr),
(70) The Powerful (al-Muqtadir)
(71) The Promoter (al-Muqaddim)
(72) The Postponer (al-Mu'akhkhir)
(73) The First (al-Awwal),

(74) The Last (al-Ākhir),
(75) The Manifest (al-Ẓāhir)
(76) The Hidden (al-Bāṭin);
(77) The Governor (al-Wālī)
(78) The Exalted (al-Muta'ālī)
(79) The Source of All Goodness (al-Barr)
(80) The Acceptor of Repentance (al-Tawwāb)
(81) The Avenger (al-Muntaqim)
(82) The Pardoner (al-'Afū);
(83) The Clement (al-Ra'ūf)
(84) King of Absolute Sovereignty (Mālik al-Mulk)
(85) Lord of Majesty and Generosity (Dhū 'l-Jalāl wa'l-Ikrām)
(86) The Equitable (al-Muqit)
(87) The Gatherer (al-Jāmi')
(88) The Rich (al-Ghanī),
(89) The Enricher (al-Mughnī)
(90) The Protector (al-Māni')
(91) The Punisher (al-Ḍārr),
(92) the Creator of the Beneficial (al-Nāfi')
(93) The Light (al-Nūr)
(94) The Guide (al-Hādī)
(95) The Originator (al-Badī')
(96) The Everlasting (al-Bāqī)
(97) The Inheritor (al-Wārith)
(98) The Right in Guidance (al-Rashīd)
(99) The Patient (al-Ṣabur)

ALLAH

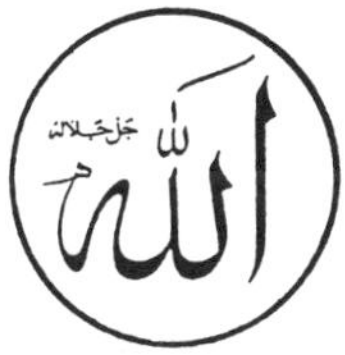

"He is God; there is no god but He...." (59:22)

God is unique in terms of true Being. No other being can be said to exist 'of itself'. In fact, *"Everything perishes except His Presence (Face)"* (28:88). It is probable that the name Allah occurs to indicate the Absolute in the same way that proper nouns denote particular things. Everything that can be said, however, in respect of the origin of the word is from the human point of view, that is, relative and arbitrary.

As God breathed His Spirit on the human form it can aspire to actualize God's Qualities but the possibility of this occurring is limited and relative to our own natural disposition—which God gave us—and the extent of our directing our motivations and perceptions towards this goal. However, gaining knowledge of God's Most Beautiful Names and assuming them as noble or praiseworthy character traits whatever possible makes us in no way comparable to God's likeness. The Quran clearly states, *"Naught is as His likeness"* (16:74) nor should one consider that sharing in every quality means a likeness. Likeness is defined as sharing in a specific thing and in essence. A horse and a human being may both be swift but their likeness ends here.

The meaning of the name God is so specific that it is inconceivable that there could be any sharing of the Name whether it be metaphorically or literally. In view of this, the rest of the Names are described as being the Names of God and are defined in relation to God. One may say that the Patient, the Compeller, and the Sovereign are among the Names of God but one cannot say that God is one of the Names of the Patient, the

Compeller, the Sovereign. This is because the Name Allah, God, is more indicative of the true nature of the meaning of divinity and is, therefore, more specific. As a result, one dispenses with trying to define it by something else whereas the other Names are defined in relationship to the Name God. As the Quran says, "*Do you know of any other that can be named with His Name*?" (19:65)

1 Al-Raḥmān: The Merciful
2 Al-Raḥīm: The Compassionate

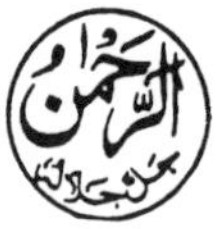

Humanity
Balanced
W/E: 298

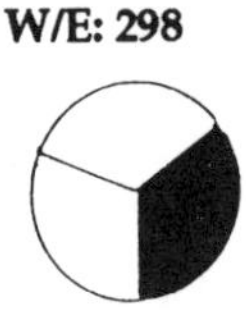

"*In the Name of God, the Merciful (al-Raḥmān), the Compassionate (al-Rahīm)....*" (1:1)

The Merciful and the Compassionate are qualities derived from *raḥamā* (mercy). The concept of mercy requires that there be an object of mercy, someone or something in need. The needs of the needy are satisfied through the Merciful without any intention, choosing, willing, or asking by the needy one.

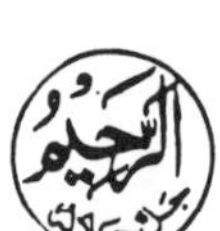

Humanity
Balanced
W/E: 258

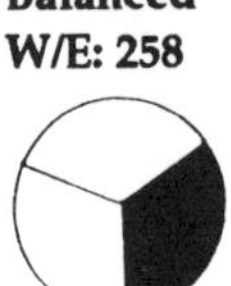

The mercy of the Merciful is perfect in the sense that God not only wills the satisfaction of the needs of the needy, which shows concern, but actually satisfies them. The Merciful is all-inclusive in that mercy is extended to the worthy and the unworthy alike and includes all their needs. There is a Tradition where the Messenger says,"God Most High has one hundred portions of mercy. He has given only one portion to the universe and that God has divided among all of creation." The feeling of mercy and compassion that God's creatures feel for each other is from this. The other ninety-nine portions are reserved for the Day of Judgment when God will bestow it upon the believers. The Quran says, "*My mercy embraces everything*" (7:156).

A distinction should be made between the

meanings of the two qualities of the Merciful and the Compassionate. The basic meaning to be understood from the Merciful is a kind of mercy which is beyond the reach of human potential and provides the needs for the *nafs* or soul for all creatures in this world regardless of their worthiness. The Compassionate, on the other hand, is the quality that God manifests to the believers, "*He is compassionate to the believers*" (33:43). God shows compassion towards those who use their free will to choose His way in order to be saved in the Hereafter. This is why it is said God is compassionate towards His believers.

3 Al-Malik: The Sovereign

"*So high exalted be God, the Sovereign (al-Malik)...*" (20:114).

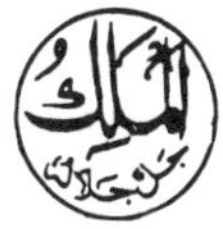

Self
W/E: 90
Cold

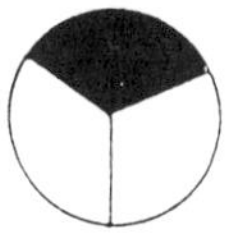

The Sovereign is the quality of being independent of all existing things while everything in existence is dependent upon it. Nothing can exist without God whether it be in respect of essence, qualities, existence, or continued being *(baqā')*. Each and every thing derives its being from God or from something which is derived from God. Everything other than God is subject to God in respect to both its qualities and essence. But God has no need for anything. God, indeed, is the Sovereign in the absolute sense. In the sense of incomparability, God is absolutely independent of us. As an active quality, everything else is dependent upon God. God's kingdom consists of all possible things, including human beings. "*To Him belongs the kingdom of the heavens and the earth*" (2:107). The Messenger said, "God is the Lord and Sovereign of everything."

4 Al-Quddūs: The Holy

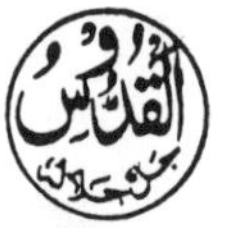

Self
W: 410
E: 170
Cold

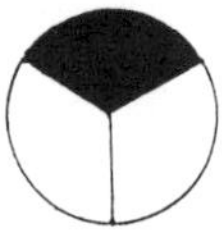

"All that is in the heavens and the earth magnifies God, the Sovereign, the Holy (al-Quddūs)" (62:1).

The Holy is God's quality of being above every description of which human perception can perceive. It is beyond what the imagination can grasp. Even the innermost consciousness cannot pervade and thereby have an understanding of the Holy, the noble character trait manifested by Prophet Jesus to raise the dead to life. It is a quality unique unto God alone for it is to be without blemish, shortcoming, or weakness.

5 Al-Salām: The Flawless

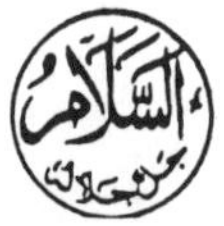

Self
W: 371
E: 131
Hot

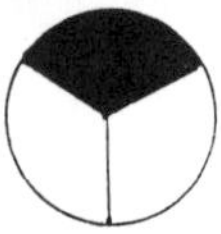

"*...the Flawless (al-Salām)...*" (59:23)

The Flawless is God's quality of lacking all imperfection or any trace of deficiency. There is no perfect, unimpaired state of being in existence except that which is ascribed to and emanates from God. The actions of the Flawless are free from absolute negative or base actions. Absolute evil is evil desired for its own sake and not for a greater good resulting from it. There is no natural evil in existence which has this description. The Flawless persists unfaltering, uninterrupted until eternity. In terms of as active quality, *as-Salām* is the giver of peace and salvation at the beginning of the creation and at the time of the resurrection. Pronouncing the blessing of peace, '*as-salām alaykum*' upon His creatures is also a manifestation of al-Salām.

6 Al-Mu'min: The Giver of Faith

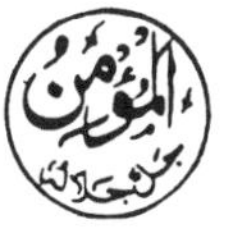

Humanity
W/E: 136
Hot

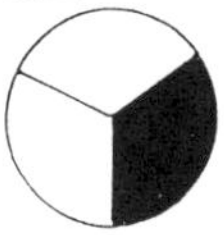

"...*the Giver of Faith (al-Mu' min)*..." (59:23).

The Giver of Faith is God's quality of giving safety and security. It blocks the avenues leading to fear of anything other than God. Only when there is fear of anything but God does the concept of safety become important. Otherwise, those who seek refuge in the Giver of Faith from fear of anything other than God are safe and secure. Safety and security in the absolute sense are inconceivable unless they be derived from God.

7 Al-Muhaymin: The Guardian

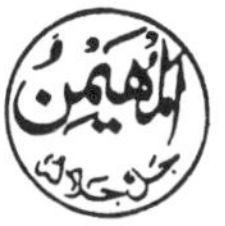

Humanity
W/E: 145
Hot

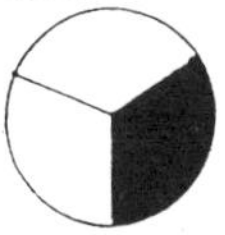

"...*the Guardian (al-Muhaymin)*..." (59:23).

The meaning of the Guardian in respect of God is that God brings about the evolution and growth of God's creation. The Guardian brings these about through knowledge, control, and protection. No one combines these qualities in an absolute and perfect sense other than God.

8 Al-'Azīz: The Incomparable

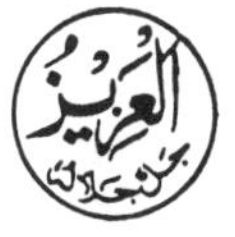

Self
W/E: 94
Cold

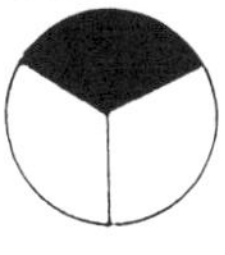

"...*the Incomparable (al-'Azīz)*.." (59:23).

God is the Incomparable in terms of importance, usefulness and inaccessibility. Whatever lacks any of these three qualities (importance, usefulness, and inaccessibility) cannot be described by the name of the incomparable (*'azīz*). Being incomparable means being rare, very precious, and difficult to obtain. God is so rare that He is absolutely unique, so necessary that nothing would exist without Him, so inaccessible that God alone can know Himself.

There are many things in the universe of which it can be said that their usefulness is limited. They cannot be called incomparable (*'azīz*). There are many things which have great importance, abundant usefulness, and are incomparable in this world. If approaching it is not difficult, however, one still cannot call it incomparable. An example of this is the sun which has no equal. This is also true of the earth. The usefulness of and need for each of them is great, to say the least. Yet the fact remains that they cannot be characterized in terms of incomparability since it is easy to observe them. That is, they are not unapproachable. Therefore, it is necessary that these three characteristics be combined before one can refer to something as being incomparable. Our absolute need exists for God alone. No one really knows God except God.

9 Al-Jabbār: The Compeller

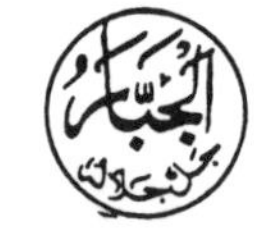

"*...the Compeller (al-Jabbār)...*" (59:23).

Creation
W/E: 206
Balanced

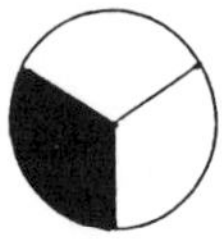

The Compeller is God's quality of being effective in terms of will power over everyone and everything while no will power is effective over It. This force is the one from whose grasp no one is free. God's Will is absolute and this magnifies God over every other being. Through His Will, God compels His creatures to obey His counseling to the positive (*amr bi'l ma'rūf*) or commands and trying to prevent the development of the negative (*nahy 'an al-munkar*) or prohibitions. These counsels are part of the instinctive nature within beings and things. They predispose creatures to follow God's Will, the highest stage of which is to become conscious of self through which the creature then bears witness to the Creator. Certainly God coerces everyone, but no one coerces Him. There is not a single person in the world who approximates God's power and inaccessibility. According to Algazel, this quality best describes Muhammad, peace and the mercy of God be upon him.

10 Al-Mutakabbir: The Proud

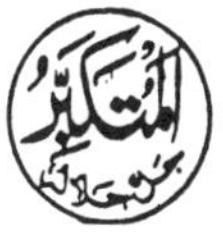

Self
W/E: 662
Hot

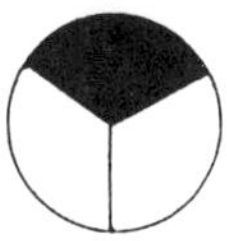

"*...the Proud (al-Mutakabbir)...*" (59:23).

God's quality of being the Proud considers everything less in comparison to its own essence. Majesty and glory belong to God alone. From this quality comes the command to magnify God by saying the *takbīr, Allāhu akbar,* God is Greater. This is pride in the purest sense of the word. It is inconceivable of anyone except God in an absolute sense.

11 Al-Khāliq: The Creator
12 Al-Bāri': The Maker of Perfect Harmony
13 Al-Muṣawwir: The Shaper of Unique Beauty

"*God is the Creator (al-Khāliq), the Maker of Perfect Harmony (al-Bārī'), the Shaper of Unique Beauty (al-Muṣawwir)...*" (59:24).

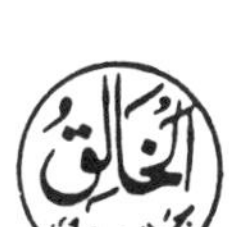

Creation
W/E: 731
Cold

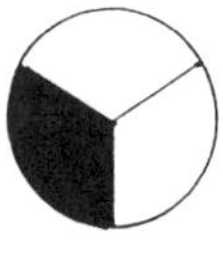

One may think that the qualities manifest in the Creator, the Maker of Perfect Harmony, and the Shaper of Unique Beauty are synonymous and that each one is derived from the act of creating and bringing into being. But this is not so. The fact of the matter is that everything which emerges from non-existence into existence, first of all, requires a planning stage (the Creator), then the actual bringing into being in a harmonious order according to the plan (the Maker of Perfect Harmony), and, thirdly, the shaper of the plan through a unique beauty (the Shaper of Unique Beauty). God manifests the quality of the Creator in as much as He is the One who plans and determines—from nothing—without any model. He establishes and defines the states of things before they come into existence. This includes the conditions and sustenance for all that He creates establishing the how, when, and where creation is to take place. Everything is given goodness and wisdom from the beginning and follows an order or plan. There are no accidents. God neither needs the creation nor does God benefit from it. The reason for creation is perhaps to bear witness to God's eternal Will of greatness and power and to see the reflection of God's beauty and perfection.

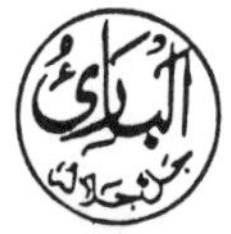

Creation
W/E: 213
Hot

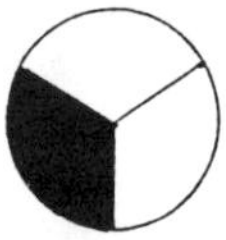

God manifests the quality of the Maker of Perfect Harmony by bringing into being in perfect harmony not only each thing within itself but with each and every other creature in relation to each other, as well. Everything is interconnected. When one part of the cycle is effected, all parts are effected because the function of one thing depends on the function of the others.

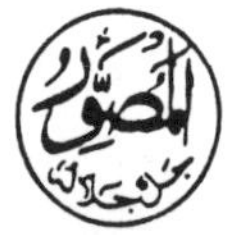

Creation
W: 306
E: 336
Hot

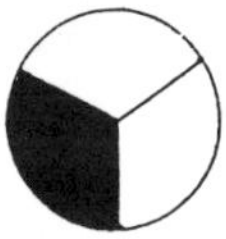

God manifests the quality of the Shaper of Unique Beauty in view of the fact that the originations are shaped in forms of unique beauty. Without model, this quality of God shapes everything perfectly at the same time that no two things are exactly alike in every way. Each and every creation is a choice creation reflecting God's infinite mercy and wisdom.

14 Al-Ghaffār: The Forgiver

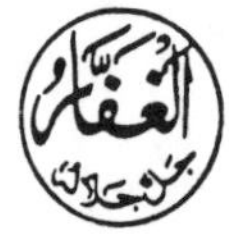

"...And I call you to the Incomparable, the Forgiver

(al-Ghaffār)" (40:42).

Humanity
W/E: 1181
Balanced

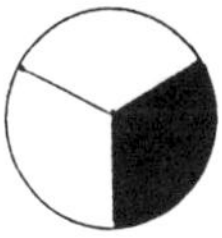

The Forgiver is God's quality that makes manifest what is noble and hides what is disgraceful. The sins of human beings are among the disgraceful things which the Forgiver hides by covering over them in this world and disregarding their punishment in the hereafter. According to Algazel, this name best defines Jesus, peace be upon him.

15 Al-Qahhār: The Subduer

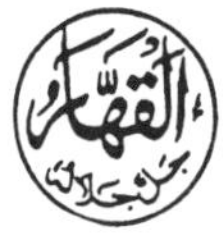

"*The day they come forth and naught of theirs is hidden from God. 'Whose is the kingdom today?' 'God, the Unique, the Subduer' (al-Qahhar)*"(40:16).

Self
W/E: 306
Balanced

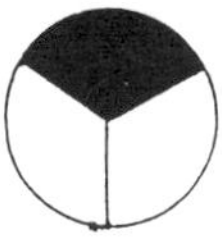

The Subduer is the quality of God that breaks the backs of God's enemies. The Subduer dominates over them by killing and humiliating them. Everything in existence is subjected to the Subduer's dominance and power. The strength and power of the Subduer is counterbalanced by the quality of the Subtle (*al-Laṭīf*) for they are contained one within the other.

16 Al-Wahhāb: The Bestower

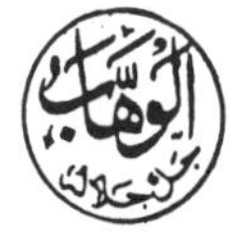

"...'*Our Lord! Let our hearts not deviate now that You have guided us but grant us mercy from Your own presence for You are the Bestower' (al-Wahhāb)*" (3:8).

Humanity
W/E: 14
Hot

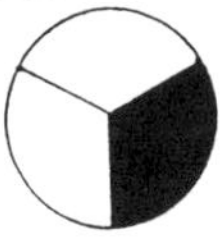

A gift is a present that is given free of thought of compensation or any other selfish interests. The Bestower is the quality of God that gives many gifts of this nature. Generosity, gifts, and presents of this kind are truly inconceivable other than from God the Bestower which gives every needy person that which is needed and does this without regard to compensation or other selfish interests either now or later.

17 Al-Razzāq: The Provider

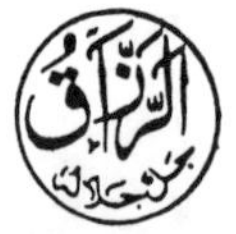

"*...And He is the Provider (al-Razzāq)...*" (51:58).

Humanity
W/E: 308
Cold

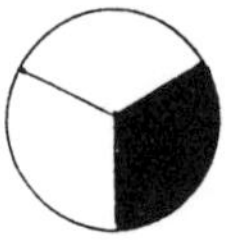

The Provider is that quality of God which creates the means of sustenance as well as the need for it and enjoyment of it. This includes the ability to gain nourishment from food or knowledge for there are two kinds of sustenance: the first is evident like food and the need for it is caused to exist in physical bodies to which it provides strength for the human body for a limited period of time. The other is hidden and consists of knowledge. The need for this is caused to exist in the human heart and inner self. It is the more noble of the two kinds of sustenance. It is a fruit which, once eaten, can bring eternal life. The Provider is the quality which assumes responsibility for the creation of both types of sustenance, graciously making them available to both bodies and the human heart. "*Our Lord, You have not created this universe in vain*" (3:191). The Provider grants ample sustenance to some and a measured amount to others.

18 Al-Fattāḥ: The Opener

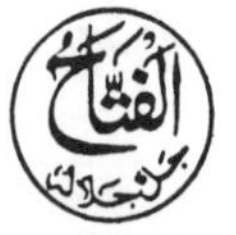

"*...Our Lord will gather us together and will in the end decide*" (34:26).

Humanity
W/E: 489
Hot

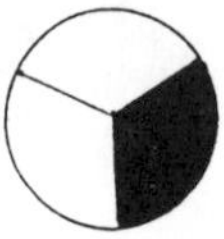

The Opener is the quality of God by which means everything that is closed is opened and through the guidance of which everything that is unclear is made clear. The quality connotes three meanings: first, the victorious who vanquishes difficulties and brings about victory; second, the one who makes decisions known; and third, the revealer who discloses that which had been concealed. At times the Opener causes kingdoms to be conquered for God's Prophets. It takes them out of the hands of God's enemies and says, "*Lo! We have given you (oh Muhammad) a clear victory (literally, opening) that God may forgive you*" (48:1).

19 Al-'Alīm: The Knower

"*...and of all things He is the Knower (al-'Alīm)*" (2:29).

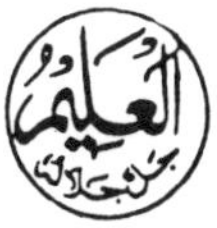

Self
W/E: 150
Balanced

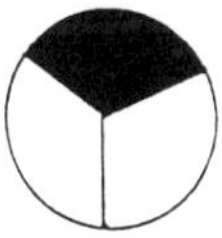

The meaning of the Knower is obvious. It is God who knows: the hidden and the manifest, the small and the great, first and last, inception and outcome, in the most complete manner possible. The perfection of this quality is to fully comprehend the knowledge of everything, including both the manifest and the hidden, that of little and that of great importance, the first and the last, the end and the beginning. All being is present at all times in the knowledge of the Knower. This comprehensive knowledge in terms of clarity and disclosure is the most perfect knowledge. It is possible in view of the fact that it is inconceivable to find one more observing and disclosing than the Knower. Furthermore, the Knower's knowledge, which is to know everything that is knowable in a perfect manner, cannot be derived from objects of knowledge. Rather, objects of knowledge are derived from it. A common Arabic expression is *Allāh al-'Alīm*, 'God knows best'.

20 Al-Qābiḍ: The Constrictor
21 Al-Bāsiṭ: The Expander

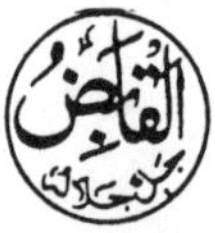

Creation
W: 193
E: 903
Hot

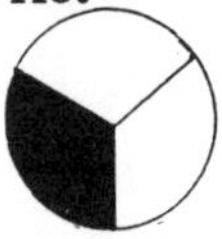

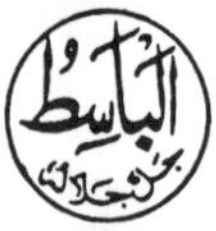

Creation
W: 312
E: 72
Balanced

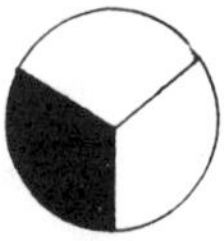

"*...God constricts and expands...*" (2:245).

The Constrictor-Expander are qualities of God that takes the souls of people at the time of death and places souls in human bodies at the time of the inception of life. The Constrictor withholds the means of subsistence and of other things from his servants by His graciousness and wisdom. It takes the souls at the time of death. The Expander, on the other hand, is that quality which amplifies or makes plentiful the means of subsistence to whomsoever God will through God's liberality and mercy and who breathes the souls in the bodies at the time of their being given life. The Constrictor-Expander takes alms from the rich and gives sustenance to those without resources. The Constrictor oppresses human hearts and makes them heavy by revealing to them how unconcerned, exalted and majestic God is. The Expander then delights them with charitable gifts, kindness, and beauty.

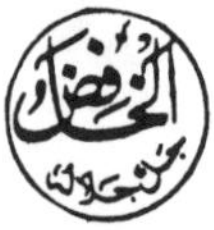

Creation
W: 771
E: 1481
Hot

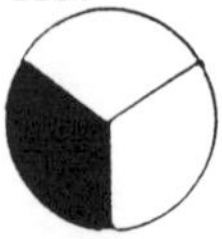

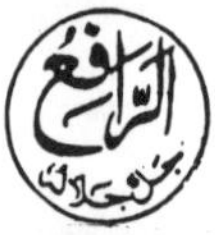

Creation
W/E: 351
Balanced

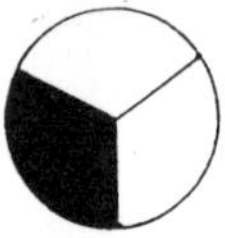

22 Al-Khāfiḍ: The Abaser
23 Al-Rāfi': The Exalter

"*When the Event Inevitable comes to pass then will no soul entertain falsehood concerning its coming. Many will it abase and many will it exalt*" (56:1-3).

The Abaser abases the unbelievers by means of misfortune. The Exalter exalts the believers by means of good fortune. God exalts believers by drawing them near to Him. God abases His enemies by isolating them from Himself.

24 Al-Mu'izz: The Honorer
25 Al-Mudhill: The Dishonorer

"*You honor whomsoever You like and dishonor ...*" (3:26).

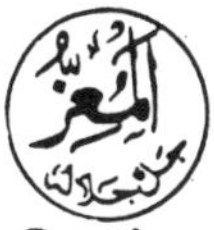

Creation
W/E: 117
Cold

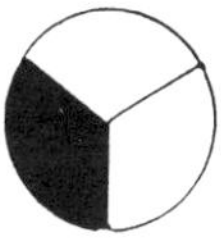

God raises to honor those from whose heart the veil is lifted so that they come to know the beauty of God's Presence, who are granted contentment so that as they have no need for the things of God's creation, and who are provided strength and support so that they may control their own disposition. God gives them immediate dominion. God will also raise them to honor in the Hereafter in terms of their gaining access to God. God will call for them, saying, "*Oh soul at peace! Return unto your Lord!*" (89:27).

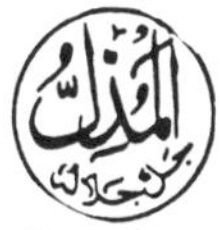

Creation
W/E: 770
Hot

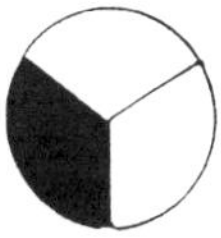

The dishonored is the one to whom God speaks and says, "*But you tempted one another and hesitated and doubted and fantasies deluded you until the command of God came to pass and the deceiver deceived you concerning God; so this day no ransom can be taken for you...*" (57:14). This is the utmost limit of dishonor.

26 Al-Samī': The All-Hearing

"*Behold! a woman of 'Imran said, 'Oh my Lord! I do dedicate unto You what is in my womb for Your special service so accept this of me for You are the All-Hearing (al-Samī')'*" (3:35).

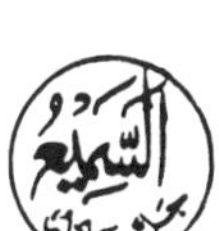

Self
W: 420
E: 180
Hot

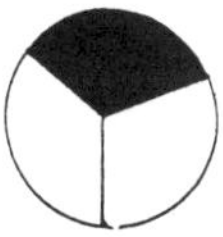

The All-Hearing is the quality of God's perception from which nothing audible escapes even if it is silent. The All-Hearing is conscious of an ant creeping on a huge boulder in the pitch-dark of night. It hears the praise of those who praise God and rewards them, hears the invocations of those who invoke God and answers them. The All-

Hearing hears without having the usual auditory channels. The hearing of the All-Hearing is not to be compared with that hearing to which ordinary speech can gain access. This hearing is of such a nature that by it the perfection of the names and qualities of all things heard is disclosed. It is beyond our imagination, free of any change that may affect it when audible things occur and above that which is heard by the human ear or some device and instrument. Whoever does not examine this view closely will certainly fall into the snare of anthropomorphism. Therefore, we must be on our guard and watch carefully in this matter.

27 Al-Baṣīr: The All-Seeing

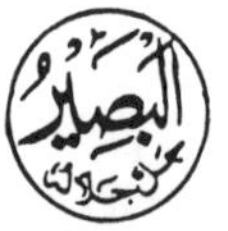

"....*God is the All-Hearing, the All-Seeing (al-Baṣīr)*" (4:58).

Self
W: 272
E: 302
Hot

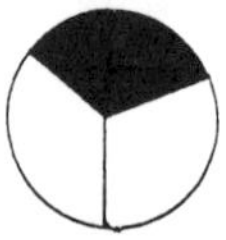

The All-Seeing is a quality which watches and observes things in such a way that nothing escapes its attention including even what is under the earth. Moreover, it is free of any dependence upon a pupil of the eye, eyelids, or the imprinting of forms and colors upon the eye as human vision is. The perfection of qualities of visible things is disclosed to the All-Seeing. This is more clear than what can be grasped by the perception of a sense of sight which is limited to the appearance of things visible.

28 Al-Ḥakam: The Arbiter

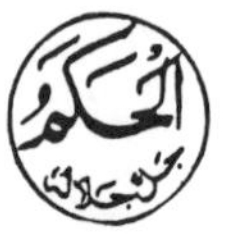

"...*Now surely His alone as the Master is the Judgment...*" (6:62).

Self
W/E: 68
Cold

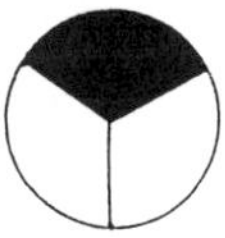

The Arbiter is like an arbitrating magistrate and an avenging judge whose decisions no one overturns or corrects. Among The Arbiter's rulings in respect to the human being are that "*the human being has only that for which he strives and that his effort will be seen,*" (53:39-40) and that "*the righteous verily will meet happiness while the wicked verily will be in hell*" (82:13-14). The Arbiter's ruling regarding happiness for the righteous and misery for the wicked is that God makes good or evil, positive or negative, a cause which leads those who practice them to happiness or misery. In a similar way, God makes medication and poison the causes which lead those who take them to recovery or death. If the meaning of ruling is to arrange causes to their effects, then God is the absolute arbiter because God is the cause of all causes in general and in particular.

The Divine decree and predestination (*qada' wa qadar*) issue from the Arbiter. Causes are directed to the effects in the Arbiter's judgment. The decree (*qada'*) provides the universal causes—original, fixed, and stable—like the earth, the heavens, the stars, the celestial bodies, and their harmonious and eternal movements which do not change in their orbit and do not cease to exist "*until the term prescribed is run*" (2:235). God says, "*Then He ordained them seven heavens in two days and inspired in each heaven its mandate*" (41:12). The Arbiter applies these causes with their harmonious, defined, planned, and tangible movements to the effects resulting from them, moment after moment. This is known as predestination (*qadar*). The ruling of the Arbiter is the initial planning and the first command which is like "*a twinkling of the eye*" (16:77).

In other words, the decree posits universal and constant causes while predestination applies these universal causes with their foreordained and measured movements to their effects, numbered and defined, according to a determined measure which neither increases nor decreases. This is how nothing escapes from God's decree and predestination.

29 Al-'Adl: The Just

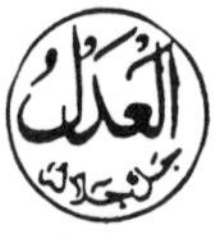

Self
W/E: 104
Cold

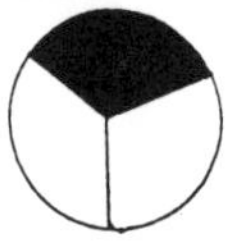

"*Verily God commands justice..*" (16:92).

Those who do not know their own sense of justice cannot know the Just. Those who are not aware of their actions cannot know their sense of justice. In order to understand this quality, human beings must have a comprehensive knowledge of the actions of God ranging from the highest kingdom of the heavens to the farthest reaches of the earth. This knowledge results where they do not see "*any fault in the creation of the Merciful*" and then look again at it. They see no flaw. Then they look yet again and "*(their) sight returns unto (them) weakened and made dim,*" (67:3) having been dazzled by God and bewildered by the symmetry and systematic order. In this condition they love God since they know something of the "meaning" of God's justice.

God created the parts of everything in existence, both the physical and the spiritual and gave to each one its own character. In doing this He showed His generosity. He also placed each one in a rank suitable to it. In doing this He was the Just.

Some of the important bodies in the world are the earth, water, the atmosphere, the heavens, and the stars. He created them and placed them in their proper rank. He placed the earth in the lowest position. He put water above it. The atmosphere is above water and the heavens are above the atmosphere. If this order were reversed, certainly the system would be ineffective.

If only our knowledge of the wonders of the

universe were complete and if only we would allow ourself time to reflect on them and the other bodies surrounding them, then we would be among those of whom God said, "*We will show them Our Signs upon the horizons and within themselves until it is clear to them that it is the Real (the Truth)*" (41:53). How can we be one of those of whom He said, "*Thus did We show Abraham the kingdom of the heavens and the earth that he might be of those possessing certainty*?" (6:75). How can "*the gates of heaven be opened,*" (54:11) to those who are completely absorbed in the anxiety of this world, those who are enslaved by greed and passion?

30 Al-Laṭīf: The Subtle

"*...He is the Subtle (al-Laṭīf)...*" (6:103).

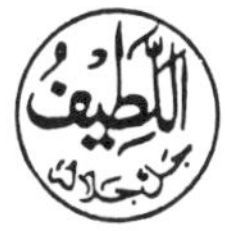

Self
W/E: 129
Hot

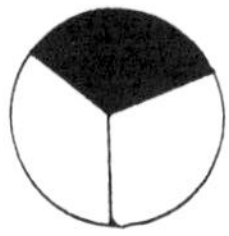

The one worthy of this Name is the one who knows the fine points of those things that are beneficial as well as their obscurities, niceties, and subtleties and who then makes them available to the deserving one in a gentle rather than a harsh manner. The real meaning of the Subtle combines gentleness in action with delicacy of perception. The perfection of the Subtle in respect of knowledge and activity is inconceivable except for God.

The Subtle's comprehension of the fine points and the hidden aspects cannot be explained. Suffice it to say that the hidden is as open to His knowledge as is the manifest. There is absolutely no distinction between them. His gentleness and subtlety in His actions are also boundless. The only one who knows the subtlety in respect of His work is the one who knows the details of His actions and the fine points of His gentleness in respect of them. One's knowledge of the meaning of the quality of being the Subtle is commensurate with one's knowledge of these things.

31 Al-Khabīr: The Aware

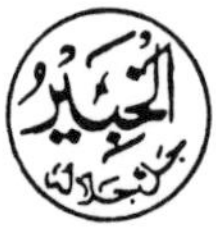

"*...and none can tell you the Truth like the Aware (al-Khabīr.)..*" (35:14).

Self
W/E: 812
Balanced

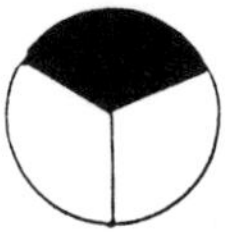

The Aware is the quality from which no unconscious content is hidden. Nothing occurs in either the physical or spiritual domain, not an atom is set in motion or becomes still, not a breath is disturbed nor silenced without the Aware's knowledge of it. The quality is similar to that of the Knower (*al-'Alīm*), both being attributes of knowledge, but the Aware's knowledge is related to that which is outwardly unknown or unconscious. It is called awareness or consciousness and the one possessing it is called aware or conscious.

32 Al-Ḥalīm: The Forebearer

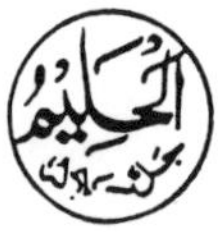

"*...Forebearing (ḥalīm)* (64:17).

Humanity
W/E: 88
Balanced

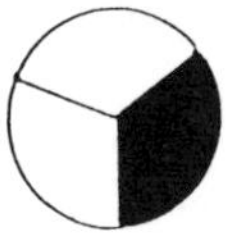

The Forebearer is a quality which shows neither anger nor rage upon witnessing disobedience and the violation of God's commands. Possessing a sense of moral reasonableness, it is not prompted by haste and recklessness to take swift vengeance even though it has unlimited power to do so. God said, "*If God took mankind to task by that which they deserve, He would not leave a living creature on the surface of the earth*" (35:45).

33 Al-'Aẓīm: The Magnificent

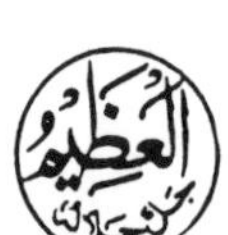

"*...God is the Magnificent (al-'Aẓīm)*" (2:105).

Self
W: 920
E: 1020
Balanced

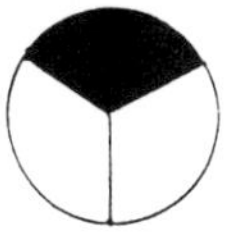

The word 'magnificence' is usually applied to physical bodies. Thus one says, "This body is great" or "this body is greater than that body," if it is more extended in respect to length, width, and depth. The Magnificent is of two types: first, what fills the eye and draws its attention; and second, what sight cannot encompass due to the extent of an objects' extremities.

It should be noted that there are also differences among objects of intellectual perception. Human intellect completely grasps the core of the real nature of some of them and falls short in the case of others. That which intellect falls short of grasping completely falls into two categories: first, that which some may conceivably grasp although the understanding of the majority falls short of it; and second, that concerning which the intellect cannot conceivably completely grasp the core of its real nature. This last one is the absolute Magnificent, the quality of which exceeds all the limits of human understanding and that is God.

34 Al-Ghafūr: The Concealer of Faults

"...*For God is the Concealer of Faults (ghafūr)*..." (2:173).

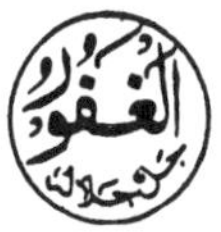

Humanity
W/E: 1186
Balanced

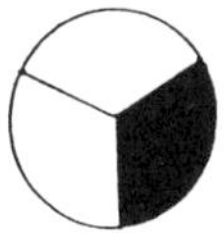

The Concealer of Faults has a meaning similar to that of the Forgiver (al-Ghaffār) but the Concealer of Faults denotes an extensiveness of a different kind from that denoted by the Forgiver (al-Ghaffār). Certainly the Forgiver denotes an extreme degree of forgiveness in respect of forgiveness that is repeated time after time. The Concealer of Faults forgives perfectly and completely and thereby reaches the ultimate degree of forgiveness.

35 Al-Shakūr: The Rewarder of Thankfulness

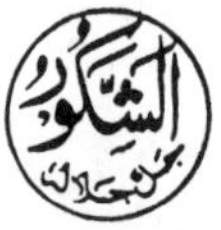

Humanity
W: 1226
E: 526
Balanced

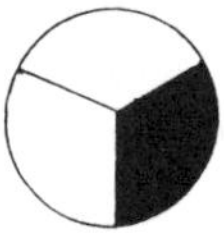

"...*Rewarder of Thankfulness (shakūr)*" (35:30).

The Rewarder of Thankfulness rewards even a few pious deeds many times over. It gives limitless happiness in the life to come for actions undertaken during a limited period. One who rewards the good deed many times over is said to be thankful for that good deed. One who praises the performer of this good deed is also said to be thankful for it. If you consider the multiplication factor in reward, only God is absolutely the Rewarder of Thankfulness. His multiplication of reward is unrestrained and unlimited for the blessings of Paradise are infinite. God says, "*Eat and drink at ease for that which you sent on before you in past days*" (69:24). As an attribute of action, it is that quality which gives much as reward for little and as an attribute of speech, it proclaims the eulogy of whomsoever obeys. Furthermore, if you consider the factor of praise to be the criterion, you will discover that in the human realm one's praises are directed to a second party, when God praises the actions of His servants. In doing this, God is actually praising His own actions, since the actions of human beings are a part of God's creation. If one is given something and then praises the giver, one may say that he is thankful. But the one who gives and then goes on to shower praises upon the recipient certainly is more worthy of being called a thankful person. The praise of God upon His people is exemplified by His saying, ". . . *Men who remember God much and women who remember, God has prepared for them forgiveness and a vast reward,*" (33:35) and by His saying, "*How excellent a slave! He was ever turning in repentance (to his Lord),*" (38:41) and by other verses of this nature.

36 Al-'Alī: The Highest

"Glorify the name of your Lord the Highest (al-'Alī)" (87:1).

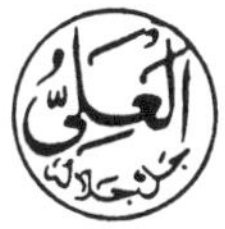

Self
W/E : 110
Cold

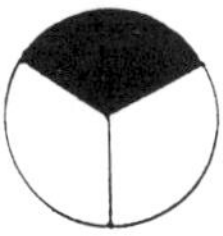

The Highest is that quality above which there is no rank. All the other ranks are inferior to the Highest. The Highest refers to height. Height refers to the concept of elevation. Elevation is the opposite of lowness. It may be conceived in terms of perceptible height or level or in terms of some sort of rational order. Everything that can be described as being "above" in respect of space possesses spatial highness and everything that can be described as being "above" in terms of rank may be said to have a highness exceeding all others.

37 Al-Kabīr: The Great

"He knows the Unseen and that which is open. He is the Great (al-Kabīr)..." (13:9).

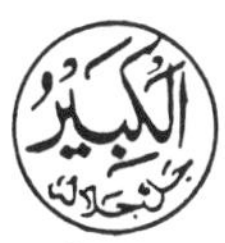

Self
W/E: 232
Balanced

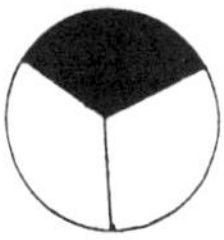

Greatness is an expression of the perfection of essence. The perfection of essence is traceable to two things. First of all, its perpetuity, both past and future. Every existent is deficient so that sooner or later it is interrupted by a period of non-existence. For this reason one says of a person who has lived a long life that he is great, that is to say, great of age. If, then, the being whose period of existence is lengthy, even though its actual duration is limited, is said to be great, then the one who always will be and always has been, the one in relation to whom non-existence is inconceivable, is more worthy of being called the Great. The second is that the existence from which all beings emanate is God's Being. If the one whose existence is complete in itself is Perfect and Great, then the one from whom the existence of all existing things originated is more worthy of being called perfect and great.

38 Al-Ḥafiẓ: The Preserver

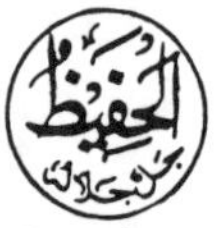

Creation
W: 898
E: 998
Balanced

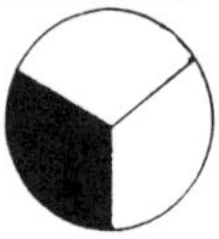

"... *a Preserver (ḥafiẓ)*" (34:21).

There is nothing in the heavens and the earth which is not preserved by the Preserver whether it be the weight of an atom or the planets in the heavens. The Preserver preserves what God's servants do of good or evil as well as the heavens and the earth through His power. The preservation of these is not a burden.

This can be understood only by understanding the meaning of preservation which may be taken in two ways. First of all, preservation means perpetuating the existence of existing things and sustaining them, which is the opposite of destroying them. God is the preserver of the heavens, the earth, the angels, and all things in existence, regardless of whether the period of their continuation be long or short, such as animals, vegetation, and other similar things.

The second way in which this term can be understood, and it is more evident, is preserving through safeguarding each being from those things which are inherently its opposite. This refers, for example, to the natural enmity that exists between water and fire for either water extinguishes fire or else fire, by prevailing, causes water to change in such a way that it becomes steam and then air.

39 Al-Muqīt: The Maintainer

"*.... God maintains all things*" (4:85).

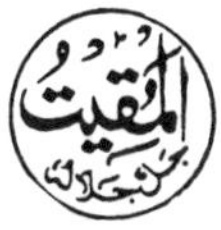

Humanity
W/E: 550
Hot

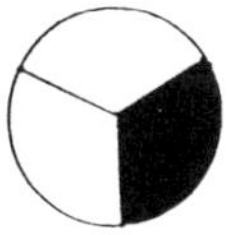

The Maintainer maintains creatures by keeping them in an existing state. This requires both knowledge and power. The argument for this interpretation is in the words of God, "*God maintains all things,*" (4:85)—that is to say, God is knowledgeable of and has power over everything. The meaning of the Maintainer would then refer back to what is meant by power and knowledge. In terms of this meaning, the quality of the Maintainer is more complete than the quality of the Able (al-Qādir) alone and the Knower (al-'Alīm) alone because it indicates a composite of the other meanings. Therefore this name is not synonymous with either of these two.

40 Al-Ḥasīb: The Reckoner

"*...and God is enough as Reckoner*" (4:6).

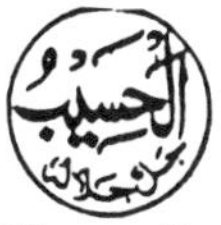

Humanity
W: 320
E: 80
Balanced

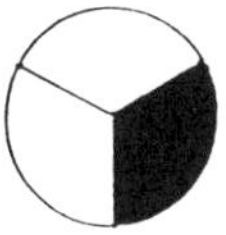

The Reckoner is the quality which suffices. As an active attribute, it creates what is sufficient for God's servants. As an attribute of speech, God asks of whomsoever is submissive to the Law to account for what he does of the positive and of the negative. The Reckoner is of such a nature that when one is so blessed with this quality, one has everything. It is inconceivable that anyone but God would have this quality in an absolute sense. The reason is that everything God created requires sufficiency of its needs in order to continue being. God alone is sufficient for everything, not just for some things. That is to say, God alone is the Reckoner. God is the cause of the being of things, their continuation, and their perfection.

41 Al-Jalīl: The Majestic

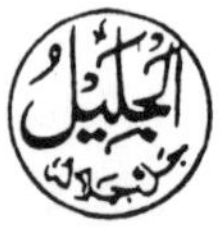

Self
W/E: 73
Cold

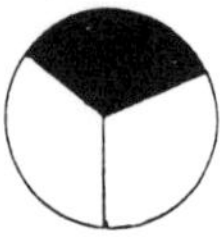

The qualities of majesty include strength, dominion, holiness, knowledge, wealth, power and so forth. The one who combines all of them in their person is absolutely majestic. If one is characterized by only some of them, one's majesty is commensurate with the attainment of that quality. The absolutely majestic is God alone. It may be said that al-Kabīr, the Great, is traceable to the perfection of the essence, al-Jalīl, the Majestic, to the perfection of the qualities and al-'Aẓīm, the Magnificent, to the perfection of essence and qualities. This is what is perceived by intellectual insight provided that it encompasses intellectual perception and not the reverse.

Furthermore, when the attributes of majesty are perceived by intellectual perception, majesty is called beauty. The one who is characterized by it is called beautiful. The name al-Jamīl, the Beautiful, was used originally in regard to whatever was visible. Then it was transferred to the inner form which is perceived by insight. Thus one speaks of conduct of being good and beautiful. One says that one's character is beautiful and that beauty is perceived by the powers of insight and not by physical sight. Indeed, inner forms are seen as beautiful by the inner powers of a perceiver if they are perfect and harmoniously proportionate, combine all the perfections suitable to them as they ought to, in such a manner as they should be combined. When people gaze upon them, they experience greater joy, delight, and emotion than those who gaze through external sight alone. Therefore, the absolutely and authentically beautiful one is God alone for all the beauty, perfection, splendor, and attractiveness in this world are from the lights of God's essence and the traces of God's qualities. Nothing in the whole of existence has absolute perfection either actually or potentially except God. For this reason, those who know God and contemplate God's beauty experience such delight, happiness, joy, and pleasure that they disdain the delights of paradise as well as the beauty of interior meaning perceived by intellectual perception. Moreover, there is no comparison between the beauty of the external forms and the beauty of interior meaning perceived by intellectual perception. Stressing the concept of inner beauty distinguishes the Majestic (al-Jalīl) from the Proud (al-Mutakabbir) and the Magnificent (al-'Aẓīm).

42 Al-Karīm: The Generous

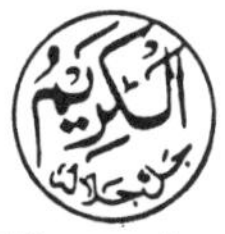

" *...the Generous (al-Karīm)*" (23:116).

Humanity
W/E: 270
Balanced

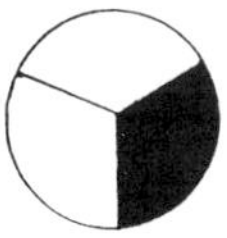

The Generous is the quality which forgives while having the power to exact retribution, which keeps promises and which exceeds the utmost one could desire when giving. The Generous is not concerned about the amount given nor the one to whom something is given. If others are in need, the Generous is not pleased. When the quality of generosity is displeased with a friend, the person reproaches the friend but does not carry this to the limit. The one who seeks refuge and shelter with someone who has the quality of generosity is not lost and is spared the need of begging. Those who gather to themselves all of these descriptions and do this in a most natural way is the absolute Generous and that is God alone. As an attribute of action, it means one endowed with liberality. As an attribute of power, it refers to one who fixes the measure of generosity and as an attribute of relation, all nobility stems from it.

43 Al-Raqīb: The Vigilant

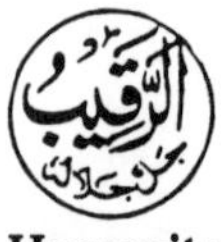

Humanity
W/E: 312
Balanced

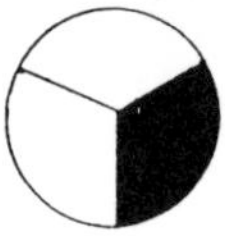

"...*Verily God is vigilant over you*" (4:1).

The Vigilant is the quality which knows, observes, and watches out for a given object. It watches out for it so closely and constantly that those who manifest this quality are refrained from approaching the forbidden. Such a one is called vigilant. This word may be said to be derived from the Knower (al-'Alīm) and the Preserver (al-Ḥafīẓ). Coupled with the consideration that it is close and constant in regard to avoiding that which is forbidden, we are protected from acquiring the forbidden.

44 Al-Mujīb: The Responder to Prayer

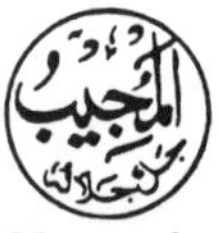

Humanity
W/E: 55
Hot

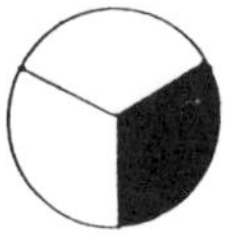

"...*Verily my Lord is ever Near, Responder to Prayer*" (11:61).

The Responder to Prayer responds with help to the request of those who ask, to the prayers of those who pray, and to the needs of the poor because of their poverty by giving what they need. In fact, the Responder to Prayer bestows God's gifts even before an appeal is made. There is no one like that except God. In fact, the Responder to Prayer knew the needs already in eternity and therefore planned the causes necessary to satisfy existing needs by creating food and nourishment and facilitating the causes and the instruments which made all of these requirements possible.

45 Al-Wāsi': The Vast

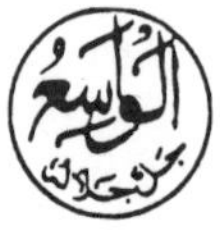

"*To God belongs the East and the West. Whichever way you turn, there is the Presence of God for God is Vast (wāsi')..*" (2:115).

Self
W: 377
E: 137
Balanced

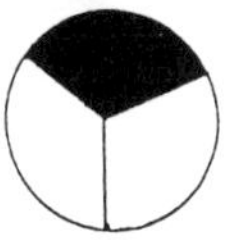

The Vast refers to expansiveness. Sometimes expansiveness is related to knowledge, as it is extensive and embraces a great number of things that are known. At other times it is related to charity and widespread blessings. But no matter how it is understood and to what it is applied, the absolute Vast is God. If one contemplates God's knowledge, one knows that the sea of God's knowledge has no shore. Rather the seas of His knowledge would be depleted if they were used as ink for His words. Furthermore, if one were to contemplate His beneficence and blessings, one would know that there is no end to what God can do. Every other expansiveness, even if it be great, ultimately reaches its limit. That which does not reach such a limit is more deserving of the name expansiveness. God is the absolute Vast, the quality which embraces and contains all things, which extends generosity to all things, knowledge to everything which is knowable, power to everything which may be determined by it, absolutely and without having to pay attention successively to things because every other expansiveness is restricted in comparison. Furthermore, any expansiveness ultimately reaches a limit so that it is not possible for one to conceive a further extension of it, whereas it is inconceivable that anything be added to that which is limitless and without boundary.

46 Al-Ḥakīm: The Wise

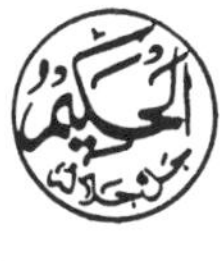

"They said: 'Glory be to You. Of knowledge we have none except what You have taught us. In truth it is You Who are the Knower, the Wise' (al-Ḥakīm)" (2:32).

Being wise or having wisdom consists of knowledge of the highest of things gathered through

Self
W/E: 78
Balanced

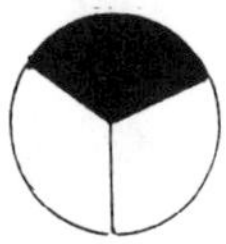

the highest modes of knowing. The most sublime thing of all is that of God. There is no uncertainty in God's knowledge nor does it begin or end just as there is no uncertainty in God's commands. God is the true Wise because God knows the most sublime things by means of the most sublime type of knowledge. Only the knowledge of God can be qualified in this manner. Those who follow God's commands will learn what they did not know from the reflection of this sign. Those who do not follow God's commands will not grow inwardly. None of God's deeds lack benefit and wisdom and none are for God because God is without need of anything. The goal of this quality is for human beings to know that there is an order in the universe and a continuity until the Day of Judgment. It is a synonym of the Knower (al-'Alīm), endowed with wisdom, that is, with knowledge of things as they come from God and with the production of actions according to what is expedient as well as being prudent in making decisions. This corresponds to the perfect soundness of God's providence in the guidance of the world and to the benefit of the accomplishment of God's decrees. The perfection of wisdom is possible only for God. God alone is the Wise.

47 Al-Wadūd: The Loving

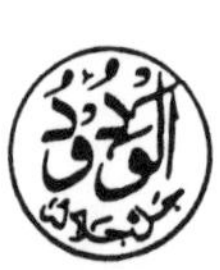

"*But ask forgiveness of your Lord and turn unto Him in repentance for my Lord is indeed full of mercy and love*" (11:90).

Humanity
W/E: 20
Balanced

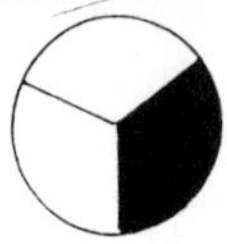

The Loving is God's quality which desires good for all humanity. God does good for them and praises them. In return, God is the only one worthy of love. The Loving is that quality which loves the well-being of God's creatures. It procures it for them gratuitously. The Loving refers to the attribute from which proceeds the praise God bestows on the believer and the reward which God gives him. This Divine Quality approximates the concept underlying the Merciful. However, mercy is related to some one or some thing in need. The deeds of the Loving do not require that. Indeed, acts of kindness from the outset belong to the products of love. Just as the meaning of the Merciful is God's desiring good for the object of mercy and God being sufficient to bring it about while remaining above the empathy usually associated with mercy, likewise the Loving is God's desire to honor and bless humanity. God's actual mercy and His grace transcend the feeling of love. Love and mercy are intended for the benefit of those who receive them and not because of empathy on the part of the one giving. Therefore, the heart and soul of mercy and love are for the benefit of the other. That is the conception of these two characteristics in respect of God. Whereas human mercy and love stem from an empathy in the heart of the one giving, which actually has nothing to do with the one being given to, the Loving is a sign of unconditional love.

48 Al-Majīd: The Glorious

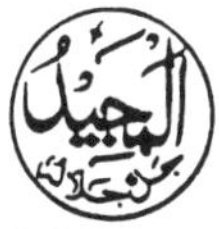

Self
W/E: 57
Balanced

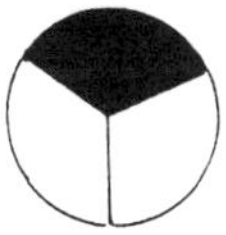

God the Glorious is seen in that which is noble in its essence, beautiful in its acts, and generous in its gifts. Even as nobility of essence when joined to goodness in deeds is 'glory' so that God is called the Glorious as well as the Noble (al-Mājid) yet the latter is a more intense form of the verb. The Glorious appears to combine the meaning of the names the Majestic (al-Jalīl), the Bestower (al-Wahhāb), and the Generous (al-Karīm).

49 Al-Bā'ith: The Resurrector

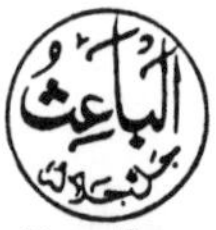

Creation
W/E: 573
Balanced

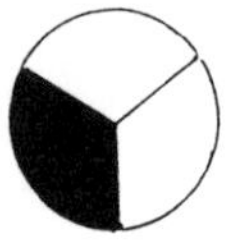

"*...raising up those in the grave...*" (22:7)

The Resurrector is God's quality of "*raising up those in the grave,*" (22:7) and "*revealing what is in people's hearts*" (100:10). The raising of the dead can be called the final 'creation'. It is a time when God will raise human beings from their graves and bring forward all the actions, thoughts, and feelings that they encountered in their lifetime. Human beings will die the way that they lived. They will be resurrected the way that they die. Whatever they plant here, they will reap in the hereafter.

Knowledge of the Resurrector is difficult to attain. The majority of people know about it only in terms of general suppositions and obscure imaginings. The farthest their minds can go in this respect is their imagining that death is equivalent to nothingness. They consider the resurrection to be another 'bringing into existence' initiated after a period of nothingness, as was the case with the first creation. But they are mistaken in this view. They are also mistaken in thinking that the second act of bringing into existence will be like the first one.

As for their thinking that death is nothingness, this is groundless. The grave is either one of the pits of the fires of hell or a garden from one of the gardens of paradise. As for the dead, they are either happy and not dead because "*think not of those who are slain in the way of God as dead. Nay, they are living. With their Lord they have provision. Jubilant (are they) because of that which God has bestowed upon them of His bounty,*" (3:169)—or they are alive and wretched. It was for this reason that the Messenger of God called out to the enemy who had died in the battle of Badr, saying, "Certainly I have found the victory which my Lord has promised me to be true. Have you also found the punishment which your Lord has promised you to be true?"

And when someone asked him, "But how do you call people who have died?" he answered, "They hear me as clearly as you do. The difference is that they are unable to answer."

Inner vision has shown the masters of insight that human beings have been created for eternity and that there is no question of there not being an eternal eternal afterlife. True, freedom of action may at one time be cut off from the body, and then one says, "He has died," at another time it may be returned to the body and then one says, "He lives and is resurrected," that is to say, his body has been brought back to life.

As for their thinking that the resurrection is a second creation which is just like the first creation, this is also not correct. Rather the resurrection is another creation not at all related to the first creation. For human beings there are numerous creations and not only two. God said, "*We are able to substitute others like unto you in your stead and to produce you again in the condition or form which you knew not*" (56:61). God also said, after the creation of the little lump of flesh and the clot of blood, "*then We produced it as another creation so blessed be God, the Best of Creators*" (23:14). Thus sperm is formed from earth. The lump of flesh is formed from the sperm. The clot of blood is formed from the lump of flesh. The spirit is formed from the clot of blood. Because of the greatness and majesty of the formation of the spirit and because it is something divine, God said, "*Then We produced it as another creation so blessed be God, the Best of Creators*" (23:14). He also said, "*They will ask thee concerning the Spirit, Say: 'The Spirit is by command of my Lord*'" (17:85.). Then God created sensory perceptions after having created the source of the spirit—another creation. Next, God created discernment which becomes apparent after the age of seven—another creation. Then God created the ability to reason after the age of fifteen years or so—another creation. Every creation is a stage. "*He created you by (diverse) stages*)" (71:14). The appearance of the characteristics of saintliness in such as have this characteristic bestowed upon them—that is another creation. The appearance of the characteristics of prophethood after that—this is another creation and a type of resurrection. God is the One Who raises up the Messengers even as God is the One Who raises up on the Day of Resurrection.

Just as it is difficult for an infant to understand the real nature of discernment before attaining discernment, so also, it is difficult for one possessing discernment to understand the real nature of reason before attaining the stage of being able to reason. And, in the same way, understanding the level of sanctity and prophethood is difficult for those who have attained the stage of being able to reason. The 'new creations' or stages proceed one from the other. First comes the creation of the senses, then the creation of discernment followed by the creation of reason and culminating in the creation of sanctity and prophethood. It is common to human nature for people to deny what they have not yet attained rather than to believe that there is something that is hidden to them. With this in mind, it is natural for them to deny the creation of sanctity and prophethood. In the same way, it is natural for them to deny the second creation and the hereafter because they have not yet attained it.

Those who believe in any of the things that they themselves have not attained certainly believe in the unseen. That belief is the key to all happiness. Creation consists of stages of the One Essence. It is the ladder by which one climbs up the steps of the grades of perfection until one approaches the Presence which is the ultimate height of all perfection. One is then with God, suspended between rejection and acceptance, separation and admission. If one is accepted, one ascends to the highest of the high. If one is rejected, one falls to the lowest of the low. By this we mean that the only comparison that exists between the two—creation and resurrection—lies in the name creation itself. He who does not know what creation and resurrection are does not know the meaning of God the Resurrector.

50 Al-Shahīd: The Witness

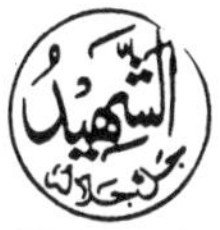

Humanity
W: 1019
E: 319
Hot

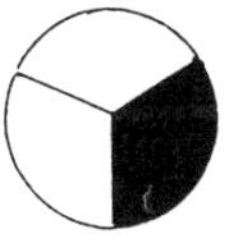

The meaning of God's quality 'the Witness' goes back to the Knower (al-'Alīm) together with a particular application. God is the "*Knower of the invisible and the visible*" (6:73). The invisible consists of that which is hidden and the visible consists of that which is manifest. God is the One who witnesses all things. If one refers to knowledge in an absolute sense, then one is referring to the Knower (al-'Alīm). If one refers to knowledge of the invisible and hidden things, then one is referring to the Aware (al-Khabīr). If one refers to knowledge to the things that are manifest, then one is referring to the Witness (al-Shāhid). Along with this, one must consider the fact that God will bear witness concerning humanity at the time of the resurrection on the basis of which God knows and has born witness to them.

51 Al-Ḥaqq: The Truth

"...*God is the Truth (al-Ḥaqq)*..." (22:6).

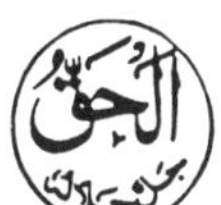

Self
W/E: 108
Cold

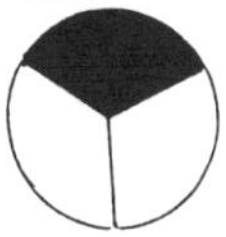

The Truth is God's quality, the essence of which is valid in itself and the cause for the existence of everything else. Everything except God is temporal as its existence is from other than itself. The Truth is existent by itself and not influenced by any other. It is in this sense that it is unchanging. The quality meets the requirements of wisdom, justice, right or rightness, truth, reality, or fact. The word '*haqq*', truth or real, is used in reference to other things, but everything else changes in relationship to something else. When that truth disappears, it is no longer valid to refer to it as truth. This is not the case with the Truth. It does not change, has no beginning or end, does not disappear nor reappear.

52 Al-Wakīl: The Trustee

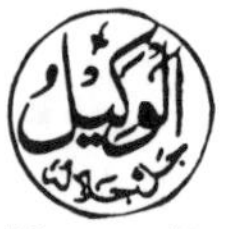

Humanity
W/E: 66
Balanced

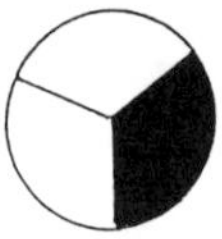

"*...for us God suffices and He is the best Trustee (al-Wakīl)*" (3:173).

The Trustee is the quality to which things have been entrusted. There are two kinds of trustees: one to whom some things are entrusted and one to whom everything is entrusted. The first is deficient and the second pertains to God alone. Those who are entrusted with things are classified, as those who are worthy, not by virtue of themselves, but by virtue of their appointment as an agent and their delegation to that position. Such a person is deficient in view of the fact that they have to be appointed or delegated. Secondly, those who by virtue of their essence are worthy of having all matters entrusted to them and having all hearts place reliance upon them, not by virtue of an appointment and a delegation coming from one other than them. This is the absolute Trustee. A trustee may be either those who carry out perfectly and without any shortcomings that which is entrusted to them or those who do not carry out everything perfectly. The absolute Trustee is God's quality to which matters are entrusted, which is conscientious in dealing with them, and which is faithful in carrying them out. That one is God alone.

53/54 Al-Qawī al-Matīn: The Strong, Firm

"*...for your Lord—He is the Strong (al-Qawī) and able to enforce His Will*" *(11:66)* . "*For God is He Who gives all sustenance—Lord of Power—the Firm (al-Matīn)* " (51:58).

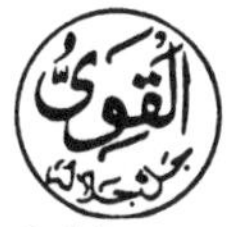

Self
W/E: 116
Hot

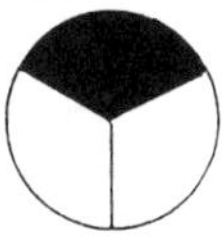

Strength shows perfect power. Inasmuch as God has the utmost of power and is perfect therein, God is the Strong. God is able to overcome all opposition because of the perfection of power. God's strength is unconditional. With the same ease God can create millions of galaxies or millions of bees. With the quality of strength, God continues the creation, protects the creatures, and guides their actions.

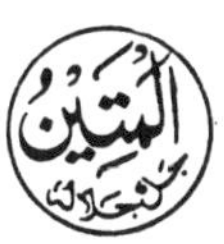

Self
W/E: 500
Hot

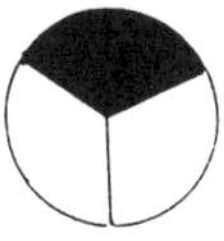

Firmness shows an intensity of strength. Inasmuch as God has intense power, God is the Firm to the highest degree. The Firm refers to the all-encompassing action of God's strength. Nothing can be saved from this strength nor can anything oppose it whether God's power be compassion for God's servants or vengeance and anger against God's enemies.

55 Al-Walī: The Friend

"*...and besides him you have neither friend (walī) nor helper*" (2:107).

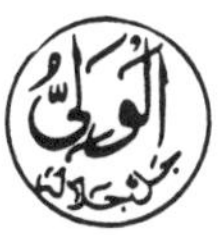

Humanity
W/E: 46
Hot

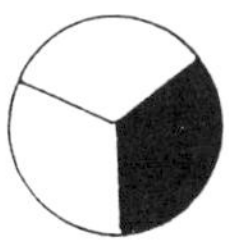

The Friend is the divine quality of helping others. The meaning of God's help is obvious, for God subdues the enemies of the faith and helps His friends. God says, "*God is the friend of those who believe,*" (2:257) and also, "*That is because God is the friend of those who believe, and because the disbelievers have no friend,*" (47:11) that is to say, they have no helper. Another verse refers to this, as well, "*God hath decreed: Lo! I verily shall conquer, I and My messengers*" (58:21).

56 Al-Ḥamīd: The Praised

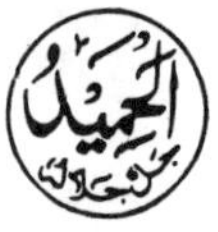

Self
W/E: 62
Balanced

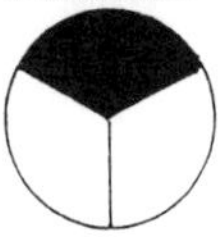

"*To Him belongs all that is in the heavens and on earth for surely God—He is free of all wants, the Praised (al-Ḥamīd)*" (22:64).

God is the Praised by virtue of God's praising Himself from all eternity and by virtue of human beings' praising God to all eternity. This fact of God being praised stems from God's qualities of majesty, exaltation, and perfection in relation to or from the point of view of those who make mention of God. The essence of praise is in remembering and reciting the qualities of perfection inasmuch as God is perfection.

57 Al-Muḥṣī: The Appraiser

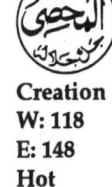

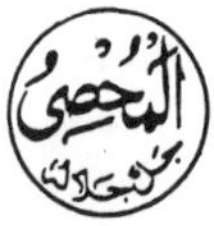

Creation
W: 118
E: 148
Hot

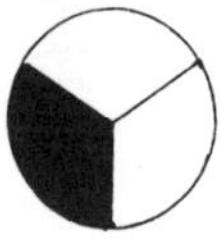

"*...and appraises everything...*" (58:6).

The Appraiser is the divine quality of analyzing, counting, and recording quantities. The Appraiser comprehends and knows comprehensively all numbered things (al-'Alīm) and has power over them (al-Qādir). The absolute quality of the Appraiser is that by which the quantity and dimensions of everything is known. Although it is possible for human beings to reckon some objects by virtue of their knowledge, yet they are incapable of reckoning the majority of them. God, however, records each deed even if it be the size of a mustard seed and the person will be held responsible on the Day of Judgment for it or rewarded for it. The possibility of human beings actualizing aspects of the Appraiser is weak, as is the case in regard to principles of knowledge.

58/59 Al-Mubdi' al-Mu'īd: The Beginner, Restorer

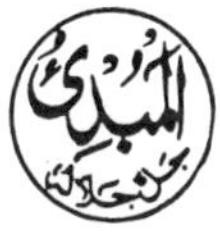

Creation
W/E: 56
Hot

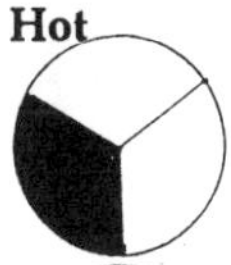

"*Verily He it is Who ocreates everything from the beginning and causes it to return*" (85:13).

The meaning of God's qualities of the Beginner, the Restorer is to bring another into being. When this bringing into being has no precedent in terms of an act similar to it, it is called a beginning. If there is a precedent in terms of an act similar to it, it is called a restoration (*mu'īd*). God began the creation of people. God is also the one who restores them. All things first originated from God and are restored to God.

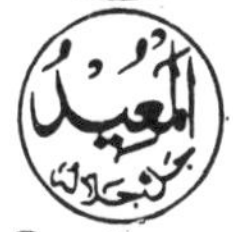

Creation
W/E: 124
Balanced

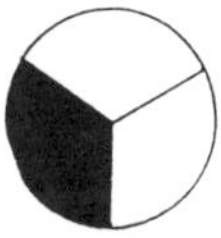

60/61 Al-Muḥyī al-Mumīt: The Life-Giver, Slayer

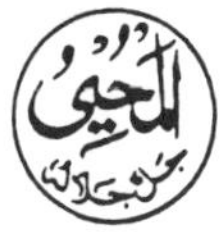

Creation
W/E: 68
Hot

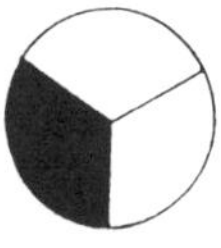

"*How can you disbelieve in God for you were lifeless in your mother's womb. He brought you to life. He caused you to die and again He will restore you to life. Then unto Him only will you be returned*" (2:28).

These qualities are also derived from the original act of bringing into being. When the object is life, bringing it into being is called life-giver. When it is death, its bringing into being is called slaying. No one creates death and life except God. There is no Life-Giver or Slayer except God.

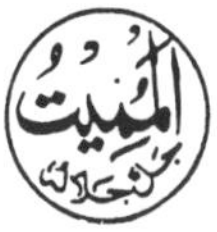

Creation
W/E: 490
Hot

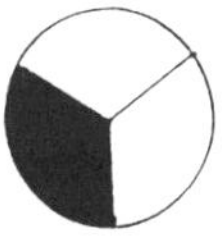

62 Al-Ḥayy: The Living

"*God! There is no god but He—the Living (al-Ḥayy), the Self-Existing, Eternal...*" (2:255).

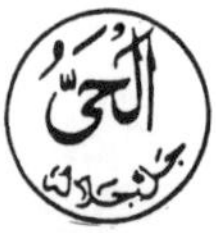

Self
W/E: 18
Balanced

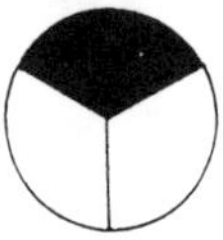

The Living is God's quality which perceives and is motivated to action. That which is devoid of action and perception altogether is said to be dead. The lowest level of perception is when the perceiver becomes conscious of self. That which is not conscious of self is inanimate and dead. The perfect and absolute Living is that under which the perception of all perceived things are arranged and all existing things fall under it so that no perceived thing strays away from God's knowledge and no motivation, impulse or action strays away from God's action. All of that is descriptive of God. God is the absolute Living.

As for every living being except the Living, its life is commensurate with its perception and motivation, impulse or action, and all of that is restricted to narrow limits. Moreover, there are gradations of living beings. Their ranks are commensurate with their gradation in perception and motivation to action, even as we have indicated before in respect of the ranks of the angels, human beings and animals.

63 al-Qayyūm: The Self-Existing

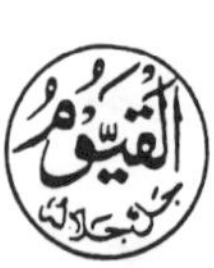

Self
W/E: 156
Hot

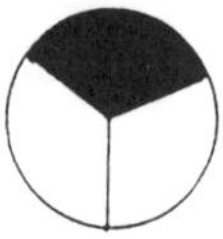

"*God! There is no god but He—the Living, the Self-Existing, the Eternal...*" (2:255).

God is the Self-Existing in that He requires nothing to exist. As an example, human beings exist or are alive because of the self within the body. The 'self' governs the body and without the 'self', the body does not see, hear, feel, taste, or move and finally dies. The body and every cell and atom contained within it are in need of the self to survive. This need is unending throughout one's lifetime. If the 'self' were to disappear even for a moment, the body would die. The 'self', on the other hand, is dependent upon the Self-Existing for existence as are all things in the universe. Without this Divine Grace in different degrees and strengths depending upon the need, nothing would exist.

64 Al-Wājid: The Resourceful

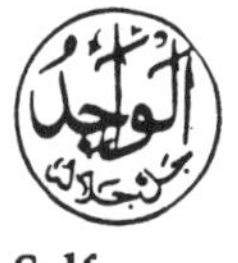

Self
W/E: 14
Balanced

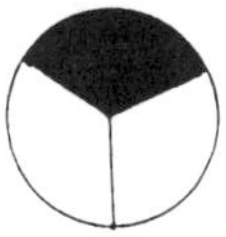

The Resourceful is God's quality of lacking nothing. The quality is the very opposite of being in need. Those who lack what is necessary for being may not necessarily be called needy. Also those who possess what is essentially irrelevant to them and fail to contribute to their perfection would not be called resourceful. Rather, the Resourceful is the one who does not lack any of the things that are necessary. Everything necessary for the attributes of divinity and their perfection is present in the existence of God. From this standpoint, therefore, He is the Resourceful. In fact, God is the absolute Resourceful. But any other than God, even if he is resourceful in the sense that he has some of the attributes of perfection and their causes, yet still is in want and is not resourceful except relatively.

65 Al-Mājid: The Noble

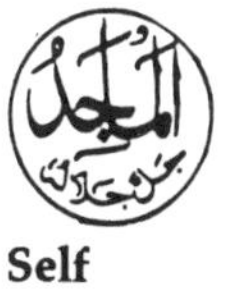

"...*Lord of the Throne of the Noble (al-Mājid)...*" (85:15)

Self
W/E: 48
Balanced

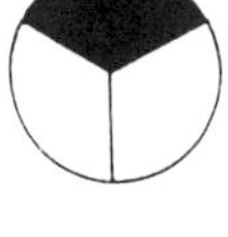

God's quality of nobility is an attribute of relation and action. It is God who shows infinite kindness towards His creatures. God has, for instance, given human beings the possibility of actualizing noble character traits and conduct. God then glorifies them for the noble character traits that they develop. Rewards are given to them and their sins are forgiven and hidden from others. Their rights are protected and their difficulties are solved. The means for their salvation are given to them. All of these are the means by which human beings become glorified in creation.

66/67 Al-Wāḥid al-Aḥad: The Unique, One

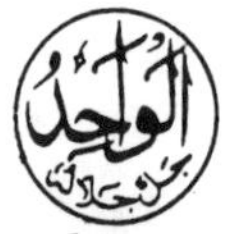

Self
W/E: 19
Balanced

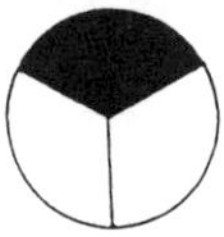

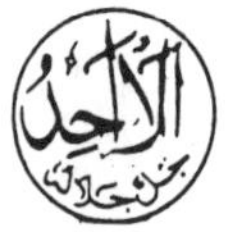

Self
W/E: 13
Cold

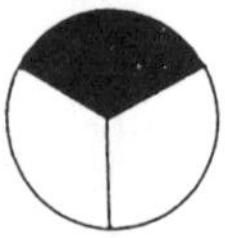

"He is the Unique (al-Wāḥid)..." (13:16).
"Say: He is God, the One (aḥad).." (112:1).

The One is God's quality which can neither be separated into component parts nor duplicated. An example of that which cannot be separated into component parts is a substance which is one in number. We say of that which is indivisible that it is one in the sense that it has no component parts. Similarly a geometric point has no component parts. God is one in the sense that it is impossible to conceive of division in respect of essence, attributes, actions, or justice. All the qualities of God are but Signs of that which is hidden within the One. The One reflects multiplicity in unity.

As for that which cannot be duplicated, it is that which has no peer like the sun, for example. For even though it is capable of division in imagination and though in its essence it is made up of component parts since it is one of the species of finite bodies, nevertheless, in fact, it is without a peer, though it is indeed possible for it to have a peer. If there is in existence an existent that is so unique in respect of its existence that it is entirely impossible to conceive of another sharing in its existence, then such an existent is the absolute Unique eternally and forever. The Unique reflects unity in multiplicity.

68 Al-Ṣamad: The Eternal

"*...God, the Eternal (al-Ṣamad)...*" (112:2)

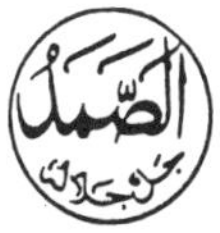

Self
W: 104
E: 134
Hot

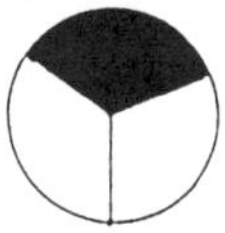

God's quality of the Eternal is one to which we turn for ours needs and our desires and the one which satisfies needs. God is the only recourse, support, and response to our needs and pain. The Eternal meets the needs of all creatures in accordance with the need that they have. Ever-present, knowing their needs before we ourselves know them, the Eternal satisfies our needs in the way they should be satisfied. This may not be the way that we want our needs to be satisfied but we should know that God is the absolute Eternal and, therefore, we should be thankful for however God meets our needs. Even if we were not to ask God to meet our needs, the Eternal would satisfy our needs. As the Quran says, "*They say: 'Why is not a Sign sent down to him from his Lord?' Say: 'God cetainly has the power to send down a sign but most of them understand not'*" (6:37). However, God has said that He loves His servants who respond to His commands with joy and pleasure and who are thankful to God.

69/70 Al-Qādir al-Muqtadir: The Able, Powerful

"*See they not that God Who created the heavens and the earth is able to create the like of them anew?*" (17:99). "*It is only God Who is powerful*" (18:45).

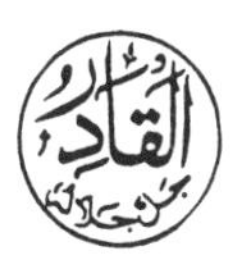

Self
W/E: 305
Cold

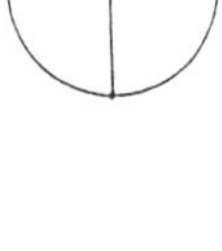

The meaning of these two qualities is "to possesses power" but the Powerful has this to a greater extent than the Able. Power refers to the principle by means of which a thing comes into being according to a pre-determined plan of will and knowledge and in agreement with them. The Able has ability which is infinite. It is God's Will alone which causes things to happen. The universe God creates reflects God's power. It is created by God when God says "*'Be!' and it is.*" The Able is the quality by which God does what God Wills to do and if God so Wills, He does not do it. It is not a part of the condition that one should inevitably will to do something and then exercise His power. Thus God is able to cause the resurrection now because God would effect it if God wished to do so. But if God does not effect it, it is because God does not wish it. God does not wish it because of the knowledge of the fixing of its appointed time and span but this does not detract from God's power to do so. The absolute able is the quality which creates every existent by Himself, independent of the assistance of another.

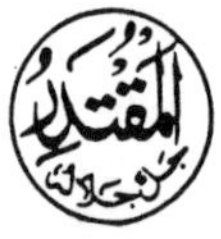

Creation
W/E: 744
Cold

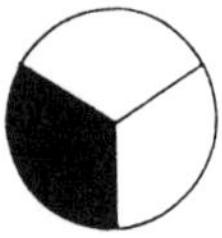

Through the Sign the Powerful, God not only creates all power but has total control over it, as well. Through this control, God is able to create what He wills and control it. Everything is in need of this power. If God Wills, God can strengthen the weak and if God Wills, God can weaken the strong. God's will strengthens those who follow His commands by giving them wisdom, patience, and perseverance and weakens those who follow their own ego by increasing their ambition, forgetfulness, self-confidence, and seeking of pleasures. In defense of God's servants, God discloses Himself through the Able, the Powerful.

71/72 Al-Muqaddim al-Mu'akhkhir: The Promoter, Postponer

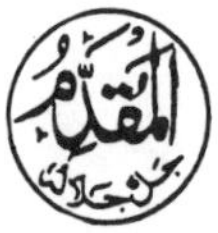

"*...I (God) had already in advance sent you warning...*" *(50:28)*. "*If We delay the penalty...*" (11:8).

Creation
W/E: 184
Cold

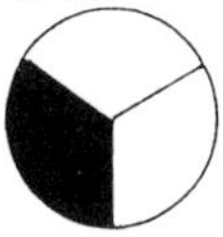

The Promoter, Postponer causes some to be drawn near to God and others to be distant from God. Those whom God has caused to be near, God has advanced and those whom God has caused to be distant, God has removed. God has advanced His Prophets and His friends by drawing them near to Him and guiding them. God has caused His enemies to be distant by separating them from Himself and by placing a veil between Himself and them.

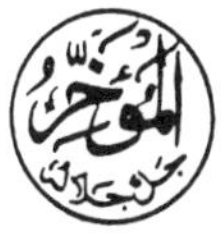

Creation
W/E: 846
Balanced

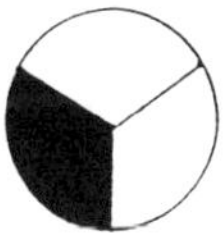

What is intended by God is both advancement and retardation in respect of rank. There is in these qualities an indication that the one who takes the place of precedence does not do so by virtue of his knowledge and work; rather does he reach this position through God sending him forward. The same is true of the one who is put back. This is made clear by the saying of God, "*Lo, those unto whom kindness has gone forth before from Us, they will be far removed from thence,*" (21:101) and His saying, "*And if We had so willed, We would have given every soul its guidance, but the word from Me concerning evil doers took effect: that I will fill hell*" (32:13).

73/74 Al-Awwal al-Ākhir: The First, Last

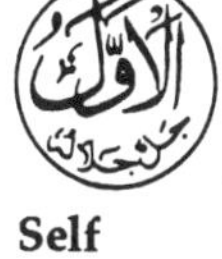

Self
W/E: 37
Hot

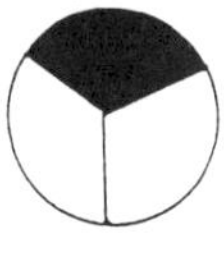

"*He is the First (al-Awwal) and the Last (al-Ākhir)...*" (57:3).

We should know that that which is first is first in relation to something and that which is last is last in relation to something. These two are opposites. It is inconceivable that one thing can be both first and last in the same respect and in relation to the same thing. Rather when we observe the order of existence as such and observe the chain of the ordered existents, then we must know that God is first in relation to them since each and every existent acquires its existence from God.

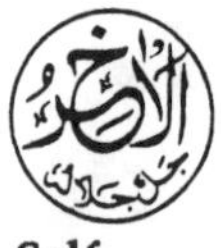

Self
W/E: 801
Cold

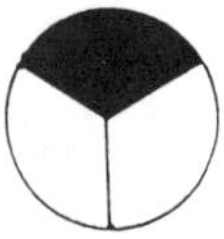

As for God, God exists by means of His own essence and has not derived His existence from another. At the same time, no matter how much we consider the order or progression and observe the gradations in standing of those who are moving towards God, we must conclude that God is the Last. For God is the ultimate to which the grades of the "knowing ones," mystics, ascend. Every knowledge that is attained before the knowledge of God is a step towards the knowledge of God. The ultimate knowledge is the knowledge of God. God is last in relation to the progression mentioned above and first in relation to existence. From God is the beginning, first of all, and to God is the return and result, last of all.

75/76 Al-Ẓāhir al-Bāṭin: The Manifest, Hidden

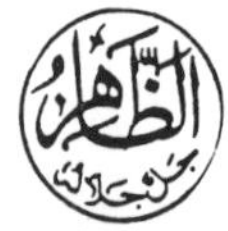

Self
W: 1006
E: 1106
Balanced

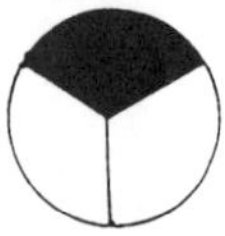

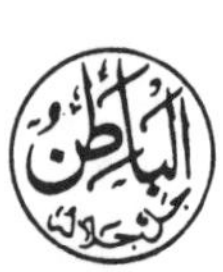

Self
W/E: 62
Hot

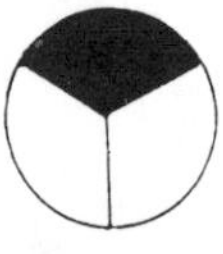

"*...the Manifest (al-Ẓāhir) and the Hidden (al-Bāṭin) and He has full knowledge of all things*" (57:3).

The Manifest, Hidden are two divine qualities among those that are relative. A thing is manifest to some and hidden from others depending upon their ability to see and to realize. For those who seek God by means of their senses or imagination, God is the Hidden. Those who seek to know God through inference with their powers of reason find the Manifest. Someone may question this and say, "As for God being hidden in relation to the perception of the senses, that is quite obvious; but as for God being manifest in relation to that which is perceived by reason, that is difficult to accept." The term manifest is used for things about which there is no dispute, things in the perception of which people do not differ. But being 'manifest' to reason is a point on which people have had great doubt. How, then, is it possible for God to be manifested through reason?

At the same time, however, you must realize that God is hidden in His manifestness because of the degree of the intensity of God's manifestation. In other words, God's very intensity of manifestation is the cause of God's hiddenness. God's very light is the veil of God's light, for everything which goes beyond its own limits must eventually turn to its opposite. Praise be to the One who is concealed from humanity by His light, the One who is hidden from them by the degree of His manifestness! God the Manifest, known by decisive proof which manifestly dominates all things. God is the Hidden, veiled by the senses, who knows hidden things.

77 Al-Wālī: The Governor

"*What! Have they taken for (objects of worship) governors (of creation) besides Him? But it is God—He is the Governor (al-Wālī)*" (42:9).

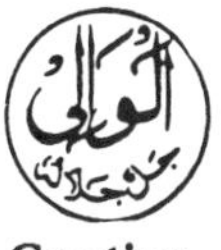

Creation
W/E: 47
Hot

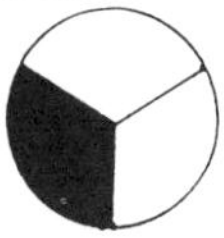

The Governor is the quality of planning the affairs of creation and assuming control over them. That is to say, the Governor takes charge of them and is capable of discharging the trust. The word suggests planning, power, and action. If all three aspects are not included, the quality of governorship is not there. There is no Governor except God. First of all, God is the only planner of creation. Secondly, God is responsible for and empowered with the ability to carry out the planning by actually bringing into creation everything that was planned. Thirdly, God is in charge of creation by perpetual and continuous actions of all the things that were planned and effected.

The whole of creation is under the governorship of God from before its creation to its end. God only says, "'Be' and it is (created)." Everything that is created is organized, grows and develops and then dies and disappears. At the time of the resurrection, all human beings will be brought back to life.

78 Al-Muta'ālī: The Exalted

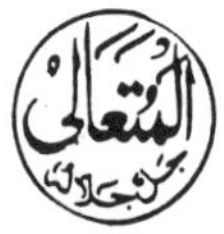

Self
W/E: 551
Hot

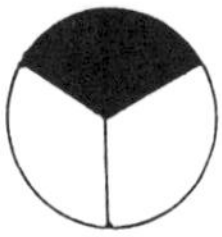

"...*God is the Great, the Exalted (al-Muta'ālī)*" (13:9).

The Exalted has the meaning of the Highest (al-'Alī) but in an intensified form. Whereas everything upon the earth evolves from health to illness, from youth to old age, from being beautiful today and handicapped tomorrow, God is free of all of these defects and above any defect. The true meaning of the Exalted is too great to be understood by one's imagination.

79 Al-Barr: The Source of All Goodness

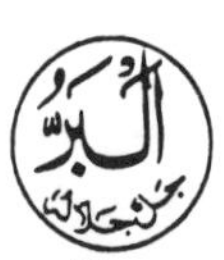

Self
W/E: 202
Balanced

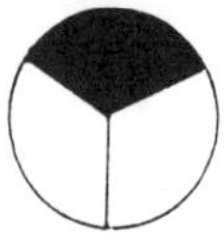

"*Truly we did call unto Him from of old. Truly it is He, the Source of All Goodness (al-Barr)*" (52:28).

The Source of All Goodness is the quality which is merciful. The absolute Source of All Goodness is God's quality from which comes every good deed and every mercy. God loves only good *(barr)* for His servants. God does not want to see them suffer yet God forgives those who cause others to suffer. If God chooses to punish, the punishment never goes beyond the deed committed while God's rewards are ten times greater for a good deed than the deed itself. The Source of All Goodness delays punishment so that the one in error may change his ways. Wrongdoings repented for are turned into good deeds. Good intentions are rewarded even if one is unable to carry them out.

80 Al-Tawwāb: The Acceptor of Repentance

"Then Adam learned words of inspiration from his Lord and his Lord turned towards him for He is the Acceptor of Repentance (al-Tawwāb)" (2:37).

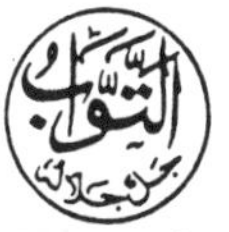

Humanity
W/E: 409
Hot

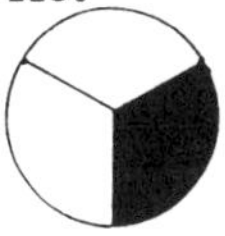

The Acceptor of Repentance continues to accept repentance from God's creatures time and time again. It shows them God's warnings with the intent that—having been made aware of the dangers of their sins—they might be filled with fear of God and subsequently turn to God in repentance. Through God's accepting the evidence of their repentance, the favor of God once again reverts to them.

81 Al-Muntaqim: The Avenger

"And who does more wrong than one to whom are recited the Signs of his Lord and who then turn away therefrom? Verily from those who transgress We shall exact due retribution" (32:22).

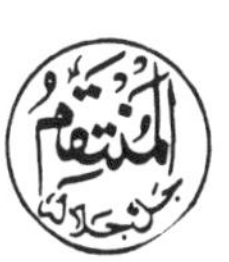

Humanity
W/E: 630
Hot

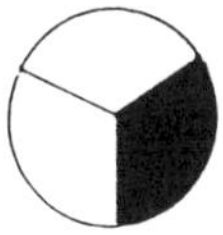

The Avenger is God's quality which breaks the back of the arrogant, punishes criminals, and intensifies the punishment of tyrants. God does that after having excused them, forgiven earlier sins, given them many warnings, made repentance possible, and granted them time to reconsider and a brief respite. This is stronger vengeance than the quick infliction of a penalty, for if the penalty is hastened one does not sink deeper into disobedience and one does not incur extremely severe punishment.

82 Al-'Afū: The Pardoner

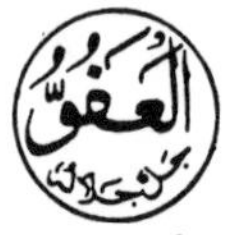

Humanity
W/E: 156
Hot

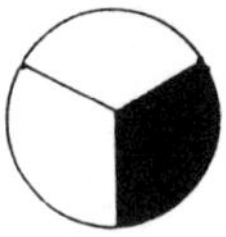

"*...God is One that blots out wrongdoings and pardons.*" (22:60)

Al-'Afū is God's quality which erases sins and disregards acts of disobedience and is the opposite of the Avenger. This concept approximates the sense of the Forgiver, though the former is more far-reaching than the latter. For the Concealer of Faults indicates an overlooking of sin whereas the Pardoner indicates an erasing. The erasing of sin is more far-reaching than the simple concealing of it.

83 Al-Ra'ūf: The Clement

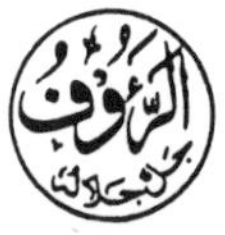

Humanity
W/E: 286
Hot

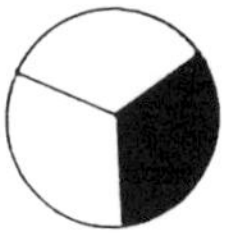

"*And God is full of clemency (ra'ūf) to His devotees*" (2:207).

The Clement is God's quality of having pity on others. Pity is the intensification of mercy. Therefore it has the same meaning as the Compassionate though in an intensified form.

84 Mālik al-Mulk: The King of Absolute Sovereignty

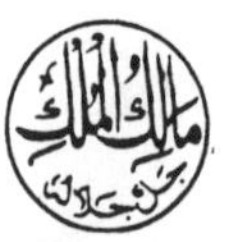

Creation
W/E: 212
Balanced

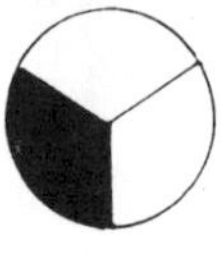

"*Say: 'Oh God! King of Absolute Sovereignty (Mālik al-Mulk), You give power to whom You please and You strip off power from whom You please; You endow with honor whom You please and You bring low whom You please. In Your hand is all good. Verily over all things You have power'*" (3:26).

The King of Absolute Sovereignty is the quality of carrying out what God wills in God's kingdom in the manner God Wills, bringing into being, destroying, perpetuating, and annihilating as God pleases. The word al-Mulk here means 'kingdom', and the word al-Malik means 'the powerful one', 'the one who possesses perfect power'. The totality of everything in existence forms a single kingdom. God rules and has power over it. The totality of existing things are a single kingdom because they are dependent upon each other. Even if they are numerous in one respect, they still remain a unit in another. An example of this is the human body. Certainly it is a kingdom for the real nature of human beings. It consists of different members, but they all give the appearance of cooperating in attaining the goal of a single manager and thus the kingdom is one.

85 Dhū 'l-Jalāl wa 'l-Ikrām: The Lord of Majesty and Generosity

"*But will abide forever the Presence of thy Lord, full of Majesty and Generosity (Dhū 'l-Jalāl wa ' l-Ikrām)*" (55:27).

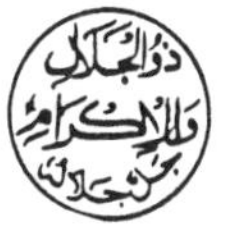

Self
W/E: 1100
Hot

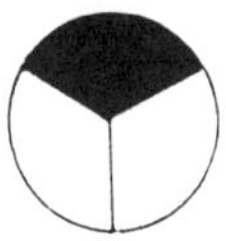

The quality Majesty and Generosity is such that there is no majesty and perfection which does not pertain to God and no honor nor honorable quality (*makrama*) which does not emanate from God. Everything perishes save His Presence which expresses the idea of Personality, Glory, Majesty, Essence, Self. The word 'Presence' (*wajh*) implies countenance or favor. "*Whoever submits his whole self (wajh) to God and is a doer of good—he will get his reward with his Lord; on such shall be no fear nor shall they grieve*" (2:112). Majesty pertains to God in respect of His essence, and honor overflows from God upon God's people. The variety of the ways in which God honors His people is almost unlimited and unending. The saying of God is indicative of this, "*Verily We have honored the Children of Adam*" (17:70).

86 Al-Muqsiṭ: The Equitable

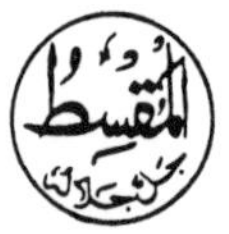

Creation
W: 449
E: 209
Balanced

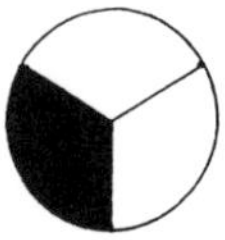

"*There is no god but He. That is the witness of God, His angels and those endowed with knowledge, equitable*" (3:18).

The Equitable is God's quality which acts and distributes justice to those who have been wronged from those who are doing wrong. Its perfection lies in linking not only the satisfaction of the one wronged but also the satisfaction of the one who did wrong. That is the ultimate of justice and equity. This is not possible for anyone except God.

87 Al-Jāmi': The Gatherer

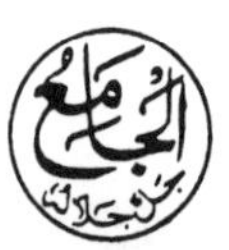

Creation
W/E: 114
Balanced

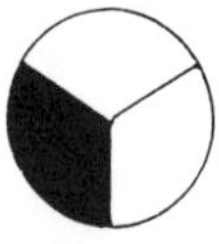

"*Our Lord! It is You Who gathers humanity together to a Day of which there is no doubt for God never fails in His promise*" (3:9).

The Gatherer is the quality which joins things that are similar, things that are dissimilar, and things that are opposed to each other. As for God bringing together similar things, one finds an example of this in God's bringing together many creatures who are a part of the human race on this earth and gathering them in the realm at the time of the resurrection. As for God's bringing together dissimilar things, one finds an example of this in God's bringing together the heavens, the stars, the air, the earth, the seas, the animals, the plants, and the different minerals, all of which have different shapes, colors, tastes and characteristics. God has brought animals, plants, and minerals together on earth. God has brought everything together in the universe, including the earth, the heavens, and air. Another example of this is God's bringing together bones, nerves, veins, muscles, brains, skin, blood and the rest of the component parts to be found in the body of an animal. Each individual cell of each part moves, seeks, finds, rejects, grows, divides, and dies. As for God bringing together things opposed to each other, one finds an example of this in God's bringing together heat and cold, moisture and dryness in the physical constitution of the animals, those things that are mutually repellent and hostile one to another. This latter phenomenon is the most comprehensive aspect of God's ability to bring things together. In reality, one does not know all the details of God's ability to bring things together unless one knows every instance in which God has ever brought things together both in this life and in that which is to come.

88/89 Al-Ghanī al-Mughnī: The Rich, Enricher

"God is the Rich (al-Ghanī) and you are needy" (47:38). "...Soon will God enrich you" (9:28).

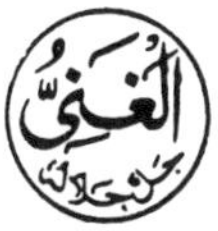

Self
W: 960
E: 1060
Hot

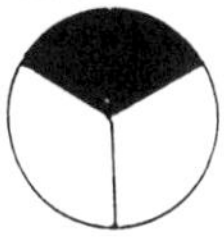

The Rich, Enricher are qualities which show God is not dependent upon anything in regard to essence or qualities. Rather God is exalted above any connection with others. Those whose essence or the attributes of his essence are connected with something external to their essence in such a way that their existence or their perfection is dependent upon another, is poor. That is to say, poor in the sense of being dependent for satisfying basic needs. Only God has complete independence. God is also the One Who satisfies the needs of others.

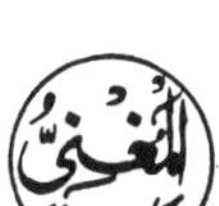

Humanity
W: 1000
E: 1100
Hot

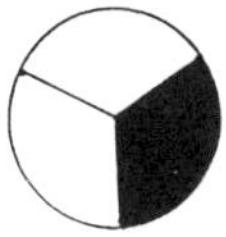

God is also the Enricher. It is inconceivable that those who are made free of want should become rich in the absolute sense for at the very least they remain in need of the One Who enriched them. Therefore they are not truly rich. Rather it is true that they can dispense with everyone but God in view of the fact that God supplies them with what they need and not in view of the fact that their basic needs are no longer there.

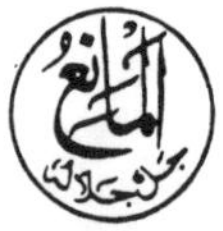

Creation
W/E: 161
Hot

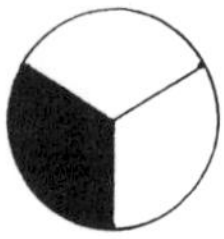

90 Al-Māni': The Protector

The Protector is God's quality which repels those things which cause destruction and deficiency in one's life—religious and otherwise— by creating causes which are intended to preserve them (al-Ḥafīẓ). Whereas the Protector stresses the idea of prohibiting and suppressing obstacles, the Preserver (al-Ḥafīẓ) stresses the idea of guarding and protecting. All preservation necessarily implies an attraction and a repelling. The one who understands the meaning of the Preserver also understands the meaning of the Protector. Protection (*māni'*) refers to destructive causes and preserving (*ḥifẓ*) refers to being preserved from destruction. Preserving is the aim of the protecting. Since all protecting is intended for the sake of preserving whereas preserving is not sought for the sake of protecting, it follows that every preserver is a protector, whereas every protector is not a preserver unless the one who protects does so in an absolute manner. In this case, the causes of destruction and deficiency are such that preservation follows of necessity.

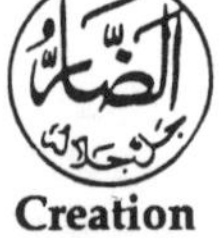

Creation
W: 291
E: 1001
Hot

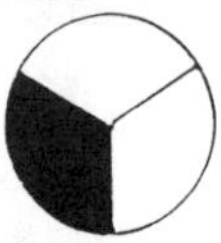

91/92 Al-Ḍārr al-Nāfi': The Punisher, the Creator of the Beneficial

These qualities of God, used especially in invocations and incantations, from which emanate that which is harmful and that which is beneficial. Neither quality appears in the Quran but belong among God's most beautiful qualities according to a Tradition (*ḥadith*) from the Messenger. Harm and benefit are qualities of God which come either through the mediation of the angels, human beings, or inanimate bodies, or without any mediation. Do not think that poison kills and harms by itself, or that food satisfies or is beneficial by itself, or that an angel, a human being, a devil or any created thing, such as sky or star or something else, is itself capable of producing a benefit or a harm or something beneficial or harmful. Rather is it true that each one of these is only a subservient cause from which nothing comes forth except that for which it has been made subservient.

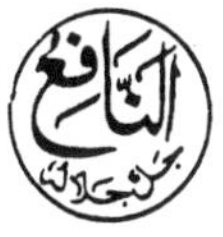

Creation
W/E: 201
Hot

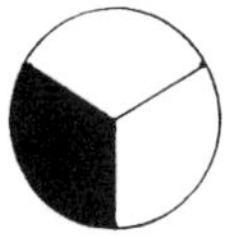

93 Al-Nūr: The Light

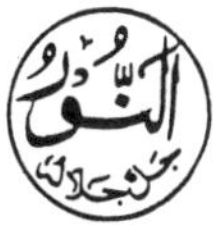

Self
W/E: 256
Hot

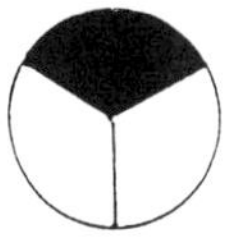

"*God is the Light (nūr) of the heavens and the earth...*" (24:35).

The Light is God's quality of being the visible by means of which everything is made visible. That which itself is visible and makes other things visible is called 'light'. When existence is contrasted with non-existence, it becomes obvious that visibility pertains to existence and that there is no darkness darker than non-existence. That which is free of the darkness of non-existence and even from the possibility of non-existence and brings everything from the darkness of nonexistence to the visibility of existence is worthy of being called the Light. Existence is a light which flows freely upon all things from the light of God's essence. Therefore God "*is the light of the heavens and the earth*" (24:35). Just as there is not a particle of the light of the sun which does not point to the existence of the illuminating sun, so also there is not a particle of all the thing that exist in the heavens and the earth and that which is between them which does not by the mere possibility of its existence point to the necessary existence of its creator.

94 Al-Hādī: The Guide

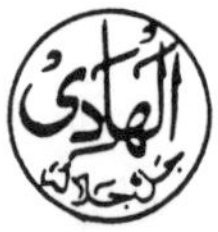

Humanity
W/E: 20
Hot

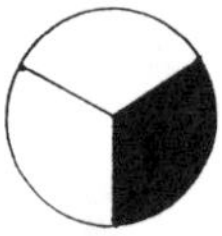

"*God is sufficient for a Guide and Helper*" (25:31).

The Guide is God's quality of being, first of all, the guide of God's servants to knowledge (*ma 'rifah)* of God's Essence in order that they bear witness with this knowledge. Secondly, the Guide guides the common people among God's servants to the things that God has created in order that they might be able to use them as their witness. Finally, God guides every creature to that which is indispensable for the satisfaction of its needs. God guides the infant to nursing at his mother's breast from the time of his birth, guides the young bird to pick up seeds from the time of its hatching, guides the bee to building its house in hexagonal form since this is the most appropriate form for the bee's body—that form which is the most cohesive and the least likely to be affected by deep gashes. This subject, which is lengthy, is best defined in the saying of God, "*He (is the One) who gave unto everything its nature, then guided it aright,*" (20:50) and in His words, "*(He is the One) who measures, then guides*" (87:3). Whoever God has guided, none can lead astray. Whoever God has lead astray, none can lead to the Straight Path. However, God creates all creatures with the ability to be guided on the Straight Path, in submission to the will of the One God. It is the misuse of their free-will and ego, strengthened by satanic suggestions, that causes God to lead them astray.

95 Al-Badī': The Originator

"*Originator (badī') of the heavens and the earth!*

When He decrees a thing, He only says to it, 'Be!' and it is" (2:117).

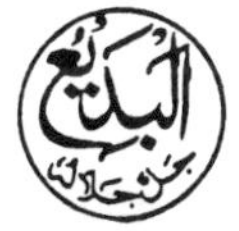

Self
W/E: 86
Balanced

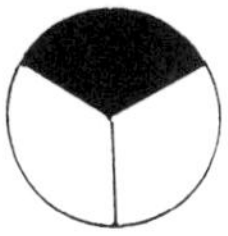

The Originator is God's quality to which nothing is similar. The absolute Originator is original in the sense that nothing known is similar to God neither in terms of essence nor attributes nor actions. If something similar exists, is it not absolutely original, unequaled, incomparable. No one is worthy of this name in an absolute sense except God. There was nothing before Him so that one like Him could not have been known before Him. Every existing thing which has come into being results from God's originating it and it is in no way analogous to its originator.

96 Al-Bāqī: The Everlasting

"*The Everlasting of the heavens and the earth* ..." (6:101).

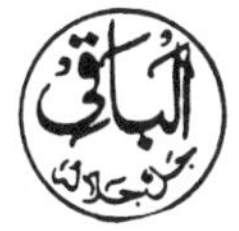

Self
W/E: 113
Hot

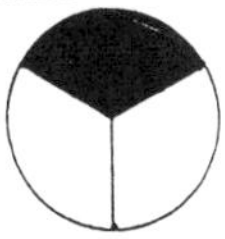

The Everlasting is God's quality the existence of which is necessary in itself. When human minds think of God in terms of the future, God is called the the Everlasting and when it thinks of God in terms of the past, God is called the Eternal. The existence of the absolute Everlasting cannot be conceived of as coming to an end in the future. This is expressed by the term forever (*abadī*) while the absolutely Eternal One is the One Whose existence in the past cannot be extended back to a beginning. This is expressed by the term eternal (*azalī*). The phrase "necessarily existent by means of its essence" implies all of that. However, these qualities (that is, *bāqī)* and *qadīm)* are applicable only in the sense that the human mind relates existence to the past or the future. In reality, only changeable things pertain to the past or the future. These are two expressions of time. Nothing pertains to time except change and motion or movement, for movement in itself divided into past and future and changeable things come within the scope of time by means of change (that is, motion). Therefore, that which is above change and movement is not included in time and subsequently has no past or future. In this sense, the past is the same as the future; passing is the same as enduring.

We have a past and a future only when certain events have occurred to us or in us and when new events will occur. There must be certain events happening one after another in order that they might be divided into a past that has ceased to exist and is concluded, into a present time and into that of which the renewal is anticipated afterwards. When there is no renewal and no termination there can be no time. And why should it not be so since God existed before time? God created time, but this did not change a thing pertaining to God's essence. After God created time, God remained as before. Traditionally, grave stones are inscribed beginning with the phrase "*huwa'l-Bāqī*," "He is the Everlasting."

97 Al-Wārith: The Inheritor

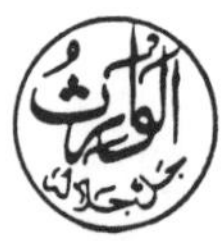

Creation
W/E: 707
Balanced

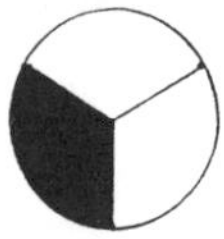

"*...and We are the Inheritors*" (15:23).

The Inheritor is the quality to which possessions return after the passing away of the temporary owner. The Inheritor is God, because God remains after His creatures pass away. Everything returns and reverts to God. At that time God asks, "*Who takes possession today?*" And God answers, "*That belongs to God, the One, the All-Powerful*" (40:16). This is in reference to the opinion of the majority of the people who consider that they themselves are owners. But on the Day of Judgment, the real nature of the situation will be revealed to them. This call (i.e., "*Who takes possession today?*") expresses the real nature of that which will be revealed to them at that time.

98 Al-Rashīd: The Right in Guidance

"*Surely you are an example of a forebearer (al-ḥalīm), the Right in Guidance (al-Rashīd)*" (11:87).

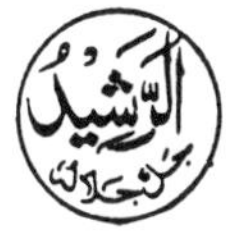

Creation
W: 1214
E: 514
Balanced

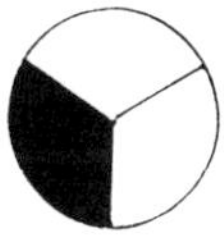

The Right in Guidance is God's quality of leading one's disposition to its ultimate aim as a result of right ways-of-behaving without the advice of a counselor, the directions of a director, or the guidance of a guide. This one is God alone. God is the best of teachers, leading creatures towards the Straight Path and salvation. God never fails in wisdom or actions. Everything God does has a beneficial and clear purpose. The effectiveness of God as the Right in Guidance is such that everything is guided by God's Will.

99 Al-Ṣabur: The Patient

"*And obey God and His Messenger and dispute not one with another lest you lose your courage and your strength depart from you. Be patient and persevering. Surely God is with those who patiently persevere*" (8:46).

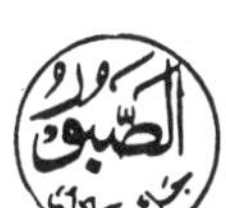

Humanity
W: 268
E: 298
Hot

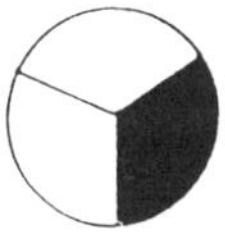

The Patient is God's quality of not acting in haste or prematurely rushing into an action. God brings matters about in a determined measure and make them happen according to a definite plan. God does not delay them beyond their appointed time as a lazy person might do nor does God hasten them ahead of their appointed time. That is to say, God does not act impetuously in this respect as an impatient person might do. Rather does God bring about everything in its proper time, in the manner that is necessary that it be and just as it ought to be. God does all of that without being subjected to a motive force opposed to God's will. God never acts with haste and therefore God is most deserving of the name the Patient.

Part II
The Process of Moral Healing for Spiritual Warriors Through Psychoethics

"We shall show them Our Signs....
within themselves
until it is clear to them
that it is the Real (the Truth).." (41:53)

Chapter One

Moral Healing of the Attraction to Pleasure Function of the Self Through Acquiring Temperance

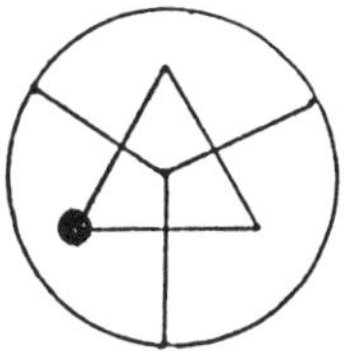

The healing process can begin with any of the three faculties but is recommended by Algazel to begin with bringing self-restraint or temperance into actuality because it is the most instinctive and its effect potentially the most harmful. It is the unconscious aspect of self which cannot be trained but can be disciplined. Temperance is expressed when spiritual warriors will their motivational impulses, which are imprinted on their imagination, to attract us them to pleasure in moderation.

Desire for food, according to Algazel, is the most destructive of desires but this does not mean that a moral-seeker should completely refrain from eating because this would be to deviate from moderation. That is, one should eat just enough not to feel hunger pangs but not excessively. The way to achieve moderation is to err on the side of deficiency. There is a Tradition in this regard which says, "It suffices the son of Adam (human being) to eat few morsels (less than ten mouthfuls) in order to keep his backbone erect. But if it is necessary [that he should eat more], then one third [of the capacity of his stomach] is for food, one third for beverages, and one third for breathing."[1]

During the time of moral healing according to Algazel, spiritual warriors should eat only when they are truly hungry and then an amount which does not prevent them from carrying out their activities. They should not be mislead by a false desire for food. In order to bring about moderation, Algazel suggests that spiritual warriors fast for three days intentionally or eat one meal during a whole day.

For Algazel there are also certain types of food which

Temperance

Regulating the Attraction to Pleasure Function Through Reason

Preserve the Species

Affect

Learn to Feel Differently

"Love your neighbor"

***" Believers are ..those who strive in God's Way with their wealth..."* (49:15)**

should not be eaten at all and there is no question of moderation concerning them—pork and any food which is harmful or not legally acquired as well as intoxicating drink. Here there is no question of moderation according to the view of psychoethics, because it implies a deviation from the Law, which is the starting point.

The second area involved in moral healing is that of sexual relations, which, like the intake of food, need to be controlled in order to heal the self. Sex is the desire to preserve the human species just as food preserves the body. Traditionally, sex is only acceptable within marriage between a man and a woman. Thus, moderation in the area of sex for Algazel can only be achieved within marriage and anything outside of that falls outside the Law. The need for sex should not be suppressed but disciplined. Disciplining it makes the worship and learning process of spiritual warriors more effective because they are not thinking about sex. Neither excess nor the deficiency of failing to satisfy their sexual desires are desirable. Moderation between the two is temperance. Most people need to heal because of excess of sexual desire. Ways suggested to do this are intentionally bearing hunger because this weakens our sexual desires or sublimation, putting their thoughts and energies into something else, or marriage, which is considered to be the best solution.

There are four levels of restraint according to Algazel: restraint of desires, refusing to be controlled by them; restraint from what is forbidden by the Law which is called abstinence; religious restraint or piety which when it grows strong rejects what is not explicitly forbidden so that actual prohibitions will be obeyed; and restraint from everything that does not lead to spiritual salvation.

Temperance is defined as the result of the emotional, affective aspects of self or the attraction to pleasure instinct to preserve the species being under the discipline of the rational, cognitive aspect of self so that the heart is freed or liberated from bondage to passions and servitude to pleasures which reinforce the material, physical or false aspect of self. It is to adopt the middle way in terms of quantity between two negative traits of self-indulgence (an excess of the attraction to pleasure limits set by reason) and insensibility (a deficiency of the attraction to pleasure limits set by reason). The Most Beautiful Names spiritual warriors will try to assume through seven stages, transforming in the process their attraction to pleasure to temperance, include the twenty-nines names God Self-disclosed to creation. The following are the stages and the Most Beautiful Names they try to assume in each stage.

Stage 1: Resolve, Submission
- al-Jabbār: The Compeller
- al-Khāliq: The Creator
- al-Bārī': The Maker of Perfect Harmony
- al-Muṣawwir: The Shaper of Unique Beauty

Stage 2: Hope-Fear
- al-Qābiḍ: The Constrictor
- al-Basiṭ: The Expander
- al-Khāfiḍ: The Abaser
- al-Rāfi': The Exalter
- al-Mu'izz: The Honorer
- al-Mudhill: The Dishonorer

Stage 3: Piety
- al-Ḥafiẓ: The Preserver
- al-Bā'ith: The Resurrector
- al-Muḥṣī The Appraiser

Stage 4: Moderation
- al-Mubdi': The Beginner
- al-Mu'īd: The Restorer
- al-Muḥyī: The Life Giver
- al-Mumīt: The Slayer

Stage 5: Tranquillity
- al-Muqtadir: The Powerful
- al-Muqaddim: The Promoter
- al-Mu'akhkhir: The Postponer

Stage 6: Spiritual Poverty/Altruism
- al-Wālī: The Governor

al-Mālik al-Mulk: The King of Absolute Sovereignty
al-Muqsit: The Equitable
al-Jāmi': The Gatherer

Stage 7: Self-Restraint

al-Māni': The Protector
al-Ḍarr: The Punisher
al-Nāfi': The Creator of the Beneficial
al-Wārith: The Inheritor
al-Rashīd: The Right in Guidance

STAGE 1
RESOLVE, SUBMISSION

Resolve or will power is the basis of all action, including the control of affect by forcing the imagination to deliberate with reason. Reason, in turn, consults with free-will and conscience before imagination sends the impulses to attraction to pleasure or avoidance of harm. Any action spiritual warriors perform requires greater resolve to become positive as their nurtured self has to be overcome so that their natural self surfaces. A positive resolve is so desirable that even if they never act upon it, they benefit the healing process. When they know with certainty that some action they are about to undertake is valuable, they develop the will power to do it and they will their body to action. A Tradition says, "The intention (resolve, will-power) of a believer is better than his/her action." That is, good intention without action is preferable to action without good intention because good intention comes from the cognitive self whereas action proceeds from their affect and/or behavioral system. Resolve shows that the self is inclined towards the positive.

Making their intentions known before acting reinforces the consciousness of spiritual warriors which, in turn, reinforces their will power. As they undertake this journey towards assuming praiseworthy character traits, by turning their heart to the spiritual, they need to give their undivided attention to every act that they contemplate performing and only act after first making their intention known. Some people have good intentions to do something because of fear and others because of hope but once they have healed, their only resolve will be to act for God's satisfaction alone. Manifesting their portion of the Compeller (al-Jabbār), they find they gain the necessary consciousness to understand what it is they want to do, find the will power, and act as they perfect God's Will.

Their resolve to the Compeller is to move towards healing by beginning to purify their heart, adorning it with praiseworthy actions. They now enter the creative process whereby they resolve to recreate or actualize the potential nature originated by God with which they were born. This time, however, they consciously participate in their creative rebirth as they manifest their portion of the Creator (al-Khāliq), the Maker of Perfect Harmony (al-Bārī'), the Shaper of a Unique Beauty (al-Muṣawwir). The opportunity is a unique one—to be born again—through healing—as a human being in the most perfect sense that they are able to do. The parameters are theirs to define. The achieving of harmony and a unique beauty, are in their own hands. Because their nature is potentially a positive one. Therefore, no matter what their nurturing process was, the possibility of moving towards the positive traits is there but the struggle may be greater for some than others. It is theirs to attempt to attain but only if they are willing to sacrifice their inappropriate desires to this long term goal—attracting the heart to the pleasures of the spiritual world.

STAGE 2
HOPE-FEAR

Experiencing the tension between various polar opposites strengthens the will power of spiritual warriors by allowing it to maneuver, to test its limits between two extremes in an attempt to arrive at moderation or self-restraint. Healing through the stage of hope and fear requires spiritual warriors to confront the natural tensions that exist within them like being a constrictor (*qābiḍ*)-expander (*bāsiṭ*), exalter (*rāfi'*)-abaser (*khāfiḍ*), an honorer (*mu'izz*)- dishonorer (*mudhill*) . Each of these pairs are an aspect of the station of hope and fear. Algazel says, "Hope and fear are two wings by means of which those who are brought near fly to every praiseworthy station."[2] Not only do they become positive, permanent characteristics for spiritual warriors, but they are the basis of all other positive, permanent character traits.

Algazel defines hope "as the sentiment of the heart when it anticipates something desirable. When the affect results from a reasonable appraisal of the probability of receiving that thing, it is correct to call it hope."[3] It is not anticipation towards the achievement of something impossible to attain which is self-deceit or stupidity. It is also not wishful thinking for something which is impossible to attain because the means for attaining it are not known. In further elaboration of the definition, Algazel says, "Hope properly refers to the expectation of something desirable when the means to attain that thing which are within human control have been discerned and only that element beyond human action has been left to God."[4]

Again, hope requires knowledge and will power or positive disposition and actions. As a positive disposition, it results from consciousness that God will fulfill the hopes of spiritual warriors if they seek God's nearness and results in action through assuming the Most Beautiful Names and other devotional practices. [5]

Two kinds of people are in urgent need of hope: those who have despaired of God's mercy, have discontinued worshipping God and those who because of excessive fear of God devote all their time to worship neglecting themselves and their families and going beyond the way of moderation. In this sense, too much hope or too little hope are extremes to be avoided. Methods mentioned by Algazel to attain moderation of hope are reading from the Quran and the *sunnah* about God's mercy and compassion and then to reflect on all of God's blessings in the universe.

The interaction of hope and fear are manifest in spiritual warriors' being a constrictor-expander, abaser of falsehood-exalter of truth, and dishonorer of the false self-honorer of their heart.

Although December's face is sour, it is kind.
Summer laughs, but also burns.
When contraction comes, behold expansion within it!
Be fresh and do not throw wrinkles upon your brow![6]

One of the attributes of the ego that brings about the greatest veiling of expansion, according to Kāshānī is rebelliousness. "Rebelliousness occurs when a spiritual state descends and brings an influx of joy and expansion that gladdens the heart. The ego listens by stealth to this influx (15:18), thereby becoming apprised of that spiritual state. Then, it begins to tremble because of exultation and exhilaration and as a result a darkness rises up. Like a layer of clouds, it becomes a veil of the light of the state and contraction ensures. The way to fend this off is as follows: At the time of the descent of the influx of joy, the heart must take refuge in the Divine Presence before the ego can listen by stealth; it must turn toward God in sincerity and devotion so that God may place a curtain of impeccability between it and the ego to preserve it from the ego's obstinacy and rebelliousness."[7]

Gathering and dispersion are like exalting (*rāfi'*) and abasing (*khāfiḍ*) and being an honorer (*mu'zz*) of the self and dishonorer (*mudhill*) of the false self. "Gathering (exalting the spiritual heart and honoring the true self) and dispersion (abasing, dishonoring the false self) are two principles, neither of which can do without the other. Thus, one who maintains dispersion (self-abasement) without gathering (self-exhalation) has rejected the Creator while one who maintains gathering without dispersion has denied the power of the Almighty."[8]

STAGE 3
PIETY

Piety (*taqwā*) has two root meanings: to fear and to be on one's guard. Spiritual warriors learn to be a guard and preserver (*ḥāfiẓ*) of their appropriate desires while they move stage by stage in their creative unfolding. They are an appraiser (*muḥṣī*) of their deeds in order to become a resurrector (*bā'ith*) of their heart.

As a preserver (*ḥafiẓ*) of their appropriate desires, when they find they have erred, they do not delay in reproaching their self because they know if they delay, next time it will be even easier to err. Their reproach is through some sort of denial of desires which are appropriate so that they do not slip back into bad habits. They preserve the limits of that to which there is no objection in order to maintain their guard to ascend from their animal instincts towards humanness by not taking everything to the limit.

In regard to being a resurrector (*bā'ith*) of their heart, "Whenever the servant's heart is tested by piety, love for this world and love for passions are removed from it and it is conscious of unseen things."[9] If they are an appraiser (*muḥṣī*) of the self and find they have not committed any mistakes, they then purify their positive disposition by further striving. The self needs to force even more difficult acts of the same type. If this proves to be too difficult, they should seek out the company of other believers or read about the lives of pious men and women to learn about their experiences.

The final step in this stage of piety is to continuously engage in self-talk and reproach the attraction to pleasure faculty so that it remains under the control of the cognitive, rational aspect of self. Spiritual warriors do this by demeaning the self to the self and pointing out its ignorance, inferiority, and insignificance so that the affect is disciplined by self-restraint.

STAGE 4
MODERATION

Moderation is "spending for one's own needs moderately"[10] in order to further discipline the attraction to pleasure function. This, in turn, "empowers the self to acquire wealth in fair ways, to spend it in approved fashion and to abstain from acquiring wealth by reprehensible means."[11]

As a beginner (*mubdi'*) and restorer (*mu'īd*) of the

heart, in their attempt to keep their actions in moderation, how spiritual warriors spend their livelihood is important. If they are able to spend moderately for their needs, they gain the freedom to acquire their earnings in fair ways and independence from material attachments because their reason rules over their attraction to pleasures and desires. As they continue to practice spending moderately to meet their needs, it becomes easier for them to be a slayer (mumit) of their false self and life-giver (*muḥyī*) to their heart. Practicing moderation leads to the next stage of tranquillity which is cultivated when spiritual warriors are satisfied with whatever they have gained through fair means.

STAGE 5
TRANQUILLITY

Tranquillity "signifies that the self is still when desire is in motion, holder of its own halter."[12] When tranquillity descends, it descends into the "hearts of the believers" so that it becomes a Sign to them that their heart is beginning to appear for that is the place where tranquillity descends. "*He is the One Who causes tranquillity to descend into the hearts of the believers to increase their faith.*" (43:4) The effects of tranquillity then are to help spiritual warriors develop to be spiritually powerful (*muqtadir*) whereas before they had only been aware of power in material and physical things. With this empowerment, spiritual warriors are able to be an even greater promoter (*muqaddim*) of their heart and postponer (*mu'akhkhir*) of the desires of their false self. Further signs of the presence of tranquillity are a greater ability on their part to relate to others with respect and kindness because of the illumination of the light of their nature originated by God (*fitrāt Allāh*), upon their heart overshadowing their idol/ego within. They become aware of the fact that "*God is well pleased with the believers...and is aware of what lies within their hearts. Then He has caused tranquillity of the heart to descend upon them and has rewarded them with a victory that is near*" (48:18) which they can hope to be the stability and constancy of the heart in its turning towards the spiritual.

STAGE 6
SPIRITUAL POVERTY/ALTRUISM

Stage six is to manifest spiritual poverty and altruism *(ithār)* as a governor (*wālī*) of the self. As Rūmī said:

They are the bondsmen of God who have written upon their collars in yearning,
"Everything lies at Your command."
Each one from their inner being has made an arrow of
"*Say, 'God!' and put everything else aside!*'" (6:91)
Among the adepts, their souls were tablets on
Which"*you are the poor*" (47:38) was inscribed
Through poverty and infatuation
They have denied themselves before their affirmation of God.[13]

Spiritual poverty is to be independent of material needs. It is therefore to be "a sovereign of the world" (*mālik al-mulk*) where spiritual warriors deal with the self on an equitable (*muqsiṭ*) basis as a gatherer (*jāmī'*) of all of their positive traits as they continue to discipline their attraction to pleasure faculty.

Spiritual poverty means "absence of worldly possessions." The absence of worldly goods is expressed in the attitude of spiritual warriors towards the world—that is, they become indifferent to wealth as Algazel points out, "A person who is indifferent to possessing or lacking wealth will not be pleased or pained by material things, and he is rich because he is free of the distractions of wealth whether he possess it or not"[14]

Being indifferent to wealth is a characteristic of seeking nearness to God because spiritual warriors are not occupied with anything but God. This positive trait requires on their part the realization that God is the Source of everything that has an effect upon them. In regard to action, they should never speak about this trait of spiritual poverty and should increase their devotions, giving beyond their basic needs to others and not striving to accumulate more than they need for, at the most, one year according to Algazel.

At the same time that they govern their now emerging heart with spiritual poverty, they give priority to satisfying the needs of others over satisfying their own needs (altruism/*ithār*). Giving preference to another over their self benefiting and defending a fellow believer, is the highest form of brotherhood.

STAGE 7
SELF-RESTRAINT

At stage seven of their manifestation of temperance, that is where the emotional, affective aspects of self or the attraction to pleasure faculty is under the control and discipline of the rational, cognitive aspect of self so that the total self is freed or liberated from the bondage to passions, spiritual warriors reach the stage of self-restraint.

Self-restraint requires the consciousness that the pleasure of nearness to God and of the world to come is eternal while the pleasures of this life are only transitory. Again their attitude is important according to Algazel because it is not just renouncing wealth and possessions or giving them away for the sake of liberality and generosity, but it is to renounce the transitory quality of the world at large in favor of the value of the eternal. It is defined as "the renouncing of everything which distracts from God."[15]

If spiritual warriors are able to maintain self-restraint, they become a protector (*māni'*) of their 'self' from worldly harms, recognizing in a detached state what is harmful (*ḍārr*) and beneficial (*nāfi'*) because they know at this point that no matter how much they may accumulate of worldly things, God is the Inheritor (al-Wārith) of it all and the best who is Right in Guidance (al-Rashīd).

Chapter Two

Moral Healing of the Avoidance of Harm/Pain Function of the Self Through Acquiring Courage

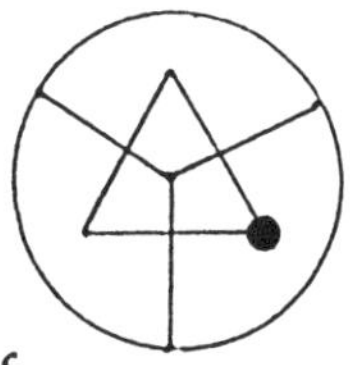

The next aspect of self to perfect is the avoidance of harm/pain faculty. When impulses are imprinted in the imagination to avoid harm/pain, this faculty is so trained by reason that its effect is courage. To spiritual warriors, courage signifies that the behavior or avoidance of harm/pain faculty or function (that is, the instinct to preserve the individual) is disciplined by reason so as not to become agitated in perilous situations and so that the action it performs becomes fair and the fortitude it displays, praiseworthy. This happens, in other words, when the self is ruled by reason.

Courage

Regulating the Avoidance of Harm/Pain Function Through Reason

Preserve the Individual

Behavior

Anger is considered to be a part of the nature originated by God which human beings share with animals, the effect of the instinct to preserve the individual. However, as the second aspect of the passions and irrational functions within the self, anger has to be trained to moderation for the self to attain perfection. As the avoidance of harm/pain, it is motivated or activated by impulses received from the internal and external senses which are imprinted on the imagination and then relayed to centers of this faculty, considered to be the heart.

Learn to Act Differently

"Do good deeds"

***"Believers are ... those who strive with their lives in the Way of God..."* (49:15)**

The avoidance of harm/pain can also act in conjunction with the attraction to pleasure function, the other half, as it were, of the animal motivational system within the self. If the desires of the attraction to pleasure faculty are necessary for the individual's life like appropriate amounts of food, sex, shelter and so forth and these are threatened by some outside force, the individual responds with appropriate anger. This is the expression of anger in response and reaction to an unjust situation and the response needs to be appropriate—within the Straight

Path—in order to be fairly received. However, if the desires of the attraction to pleasure function are not necessary for individual life like fame and excessive wealth, the expression of anger at this point is considered blameworthy and a negative trait because it is not natural anger or avoidance of harm/pain but arises because of the individual's desires from the false self or ego and not the heart. It could be, however, that the desires of the affective system or attraction to pleasure function are necessary for some individuals and not others because of their particular circumstances. In this case, expression of anger kept in moderation is praiseworthy because it is a natural response of the true self.

Traits that frequently give rise to inappropriate anger are a false sense of pride, boasting, love of wealth or fame. For those who are on this journey towards taking on and incorporating the character traits, through moral healing and giving birth to the heart within, it is assumed they have dealt with these issues and overcome all negative traits. The mirror of self, in effect, has been polished and now is prepared to reflect only positive traits as spiritual warriors' portion of the manifestation of the Most Beautiful Names.

Courage is defined as disciplining the natural instinct to anger in order to preserve the individual self. It results in the development of the positive disposition of courage through the Names and Qualities by which God manifests Self to humanity. There are twenty-six such Names and Qualities in the present Tradition and they are presented in the order in which they appear in the Messenger's Tradition on the Ninety-Nine Most Beautiful Names:

Stage 1: Compassion (Humility, Courtesy)
- al-Raḥmān: The Compassionate
- al-Raḥīm: The Merciful
- al-Mu'min: The Giver of Faith
- al-Muhaymin: The Guardian
- al-Ghaffār: The Forgiver

Stage 2: Moral Reasonableness
al-Wahhāb: The Bestower
al-Razzāq: The Provider
al-Fattāḥ: The Opener
al-Ḥalīm: The Forebearing
al-Ghafūr: The Concealer of Faults
Stage 3: Thankfulness/Generosity
al-Shakūr: The Rewarder of Thankfulness
al-Muqīt: The Nourisher
al-Ḥasīb: The Reckoner
al-Karīm: The Generous
Stage 4: Vigilance
al-Raqīb: The Vigilant
al-Mujīb: The Responder to Prayer
al-Wadūd: The Loving
al-Shāhid: The Witness
Stage 5: Trust
al-Wakīl: The Trustee
al-Walī: The Friend
Stage 6: Repentance
al-Tawwāb: The Acceptor of Repentance
al-Muntaqim: The Avenger
al-'Afū: The Pardoner
Stage 7: Patience
al-Ra'ūf: The Clement
al-Mughnī The Enricher
al-Hādī: The Guide
al-Ṣabur: The Patient

The basic instinct which human beings share with animals is so strong, however, that even if spiritual warriors are able to actualize their portion of these Most Beautiful Names within themselves, they still feel the need to be on their guard against inappropriate anger by reciting, "God protect me from the damned satan [i.e. my false self or ego]."

When their practical intellect or reason, deliberation, and discernment control their expression of anger they express courage rather than cowardice, recklessness, or fear of anything other than God.

STAGE 1
COMPASSION

Stage one of the journey of spiritual warriors towards healing the faculty of avoidance of harm/pain or anger is that of compassion. Compassion arises "when the self is affected by observing the sufferings of other creatures. This often causes a sense of forgiveness to naturally arise in spiritual warriors even if the person suffering has wronged them in some way."[1]

Manifesting their portion of the Merciful, the Compassionate, spiritual warriors recall the Divine Tradition in which God says,"My mercy precedes my wrath."[2] They allow their compassion towards the self to precede their wrath.

A believer (*mu'min*) and guardian (*muhaymin*) of the heart act with mercy and compassion towards the heart because this is what encompasses the Presence of God based on the Divine Tradition in which God states: "My heavens and My earth cannot embrace me but the heart of my believing servant embraces Me."[3] A Tradition states, "The heart of the believer is held between the two fingers of the Merciful; He turns it about as He Wills."[4]

In reference to this Tradition, Rumūī says,

The overwhelming Light between the fingers of the
Divine Light
Is safe from dimming or eclipse.
The Divine disperses that light upon the self
And the blessed hold out their robes before them to
receive it.
Whoever is favored by the radiant largesse
Is one who has turned his face from all but God
Whoever was not attired in robes of love
Gained no share of that bounty
The faces of particulars are turned towards the
Universal
Nightingales are enamored of the face of the rose.[5]

Spiritual warriors are a forgiver (*ghaffār*) of their past mistakes and errors not burdening the self with any sense of guilt. Forgiveness is defined as "giving up both retribution for wrongdoing and the seeking of reward for good done having the power and capacity to so forgive."[6] The Messenger said, "For whoever commits a wrongdoing and is punished for it in this world, God's justice is such that punishment for such a devotee is not repeated in the hereafter; when one in the world commits a wrongdoing which is covered up by God, God's beneficence is such that God does not rejudge something which has been covered up and forgiven by God."[7] They also recall the Tradition, "God is forgiving and likes forgiveness."[8]

Through compassion and forgiveness spiritual warriors develop a sense of humility. Algazel defines a humble person as one who "intentionally gives up some of what he deserves."[9] The sign of humility is that they "accept true words no matter who may have spoken them."[10] It is also said, "Humility is that you never admire yourself for your own actions,"[11] and "the servants of the All-Merciful are those who walk in the earth modestly."[12] It is to stand humble before the Truth by being a guardian (*muhaymin*) of the Truth.

Being a believer (*mu'min*) in the heart and a guardian of the Truth has in a sense a passive or defensive state yet when aroused, it becomes zeal (*ghayrat*) but like all aspects of courage—strength, compassion, and so forth—needs to be manifest at the right time for the right reason. In other words, zeal in and of itself is not a positive disposition. For example, satan showed zeal towards God when God preferred Adam (the human being) over satan. Satan's zeal was expressed by "I am made of fire while [Adam] is made of earth," implying that satan was made of a higher quality. Satan's zeal was misplaced and had no effect with God because it did not arise out of humility but rather out of rebellion.

"God is zealous," says a Tradition of the Messenger in commanding or counseling us to the positive and preventing the negative in their relations with God, with others, and with self. This is a further manifestation of the Guardian (al-Muhaymin).[13]

The Quran asks, "*Is it not time that the hearts of those who have faith should be humbled to the remembrance of God and Truth which He sent down?*" (57:16) It is to extinguish the false self, to recognize blessings of everyone who has ever blessed the spiritual warrior, and to be respectful of the process of moral healing.

Humility, then, implies courtesy. "The false self is strengthened with discourtesy while the heart is instinctively guided to hold fast to courtesy. The false self is fueled by opposing the heart while the heart tries to hold the false self back by keeping its reins in its hands."[14]

The Quran refers to courtesy when it says, "*Those who keep God's bonds*" (9:112). Courtesy is for spiritual warriors to live within boundaries and to walk in measure by allowing their mercy to precede their wrath, by being compassionate (*raḥīm*) towards the believers and forgiving of the self for its past errors.

STAGE 2
MORAL REASONABLENESS

At stage two spiritual warriors perfect moral goodness (*murāwwah*) as they move towards transforming their avoidance of harm/pain faculty into courage. Moral goodness means "being of service to others and taking no account of one's own role therein"[15] and follows the verse, "*Be staunch in justice*" (4:135).

When the great Companion and uncle of the Messenger, Hamzah, was asked the meaning of moral goodness, he said, "It means avoiding a base temperament."[16] It is also said, "Moral goodness is when they take no account of whatever they do for the sake of God. Whatever they do, they consider that they have done nothing, always desiring to do more."[17] It is for spiritual warriors to live with their 'self' by knowing their worth, knowing the measure of what they have done within ourselves, and striving to improve their 'self'. It also means living with neediness of God alone—expressing gratitude for whatever comes from God as incumbent upon their 'self', being apologetic for whatever spiritual warriors do for God's sake as incumbent upon the self and seeking God's will as righteous. It is not being easily moved to express their anger, holding back from inappropriate anger towards the enemies within—notably their false self—and not losing control when they are put in a difficult situation.

Through moral goodness, the Bestower (al-Wahhāb) gives to humanity freely and the Provider (al-Razzāq) creates the means for their sustenance as well as the need for it without their even asking. It is manifest through the Opener (al-Fattāḥ), opening the hearts of spiritual warriors to victory over their passions as they strive to improve their 'self'; the Forebearer (al-Ḥalīm), manifestor of moral reasonableness through which spiritual warriors control their inappropriate anger, and the Concealer of Faults (al-Ghafūr) for which spiritual warriors still may inadvertently be responsible so that they do not allow any sense of guilt to make them lose control when they are in a difficult situation.

Manifesting moral goodness as a moral duty arising from their needs being met by the Bestower (al-Wahhāb) and the Provider (al-Razzāq), spiritual warriors seek God's help to be an opener (*fattāḥ*)—to open their hearts to sensing their worth and the measure of whatever they have done for others and to strive to improve their 'self'. They come to manifest forbearance when they are content with others according to their capacity, to accepting of their apologies when they have offered them, and being fair to them to the extent possible. They are outwardly a concealer of their faults while inwardly being grateful to God for the blessings given, not accepting any gratitude from others for what they do for God's sake that they sense they are duty bound to do and seeking God's Will as the rightful will to follow.

STAGE 3
THANKFULNESS

Thankfulness is the next stage for spiritual warriors and once they attain this characteristic it becomes a permanent feature of their true self. Thankfulness for what? For the greatness of soul, high-mindedness, perseverance, intrepidity, and sense of honor they discover within. Greatness of self means spiritual warriors do not regard either favor or contempt, paying no heed to prosperity or the lack of it but show the self as able to accept either the agreeable or the unpleasant. This prepares them for great deeds. While they may deserve them, they do not dwell on them, finding joy in the honor and greatness of their true self. High-mindedness signifies that the self, in quest of a good reputation, has no eye for either joy or misery neither rejoicing nor grieving nor even fearing death. With their sense of perseverance, they are empowered to resist suffering and adversity without breaking their spirit. They experience generosity whereby it becomes easy for them to distribute whatever they have to those in need.

They feel the presence of the Rewarder of Thankfulness (al-Shakūr) as they express their thankfulness to the Maintainer (al-Muqīt) through which they are maintained before they ask. Thankfulness is to first recognize and be a reckoner (*ḥasīb*) of their blessings like those that come from the Maintainer and then to be thankful (*shakūr*) for them. The presence of thankfulness is shown to us when they become a generous (*karīm*) person, giving to other believers in need.

Their thankfulness "signifies virtuous action in response to blessing whether performed verbally, by hand or heart. It has been said that thankfulness represents praise of the Compassionate through remembrance of His compassion."[18] Through remembering the blessings which God has bestowed upon them, spiritual warriors are thankful to God Who rewards them by accepting their obeying God's Will as manifest in nature's mode of operation.

There is an initial and a final stage of thankfulness. The initial stage involves knowledge of blessings, the need to be thankful for them, and the nature of thankfulness for each blessing. The final stage involves spiritual warriors' awareness of their actions. They realize that worldly goods are Divine blessings and they are morally obligated to give thanks to the One who has bestowed these blessings. The nature of this is that of barter.

They understand that every faculty, both outward and inward, as well as every limb, member and organ of their body is a blessing for which they are morally obligated to offer thanks only to God in return. Moreover, they should know precisely the nature of thankfulness for each blessing.

They should know that the tongue and the power of speech is a blessing and that thankfulness for it is expressed through the recitation of the revelation and remembrance of God, constant reference to blessings, sincerity and the giving of good counsel. Ingratitude is to use the tongue to express slander, deceit, gossip, abuse, and calumny.

Their eyes and the ability to see are blessings. Thankfulness for these is expressed through contemplation of the Signs of Divine Power and Wisdom, whether through the Divine books or the planets and stars by which spiritual warriors may learn to recognize the benefits which have been bestowed and distinguish what is corrupt and what is sound. Ingratitude is the use of their eyes looking at what is forbidden, false, or superfluous.

Their ears and the ability to hear are blessings. Thankfulness for these is expressed through hearing Divine words and heeding the Traditions and wise counsel. Ingratitude is the use of their ears to listen to slander and foolish talk.

The intellect is a blessing for which thankfulness is expressed through acceptance of the Law, guidance toward performing good works, and correcting their worldly and otherworldly affairs. Ingratitude is the use of their mind to reject knowledge of the Creator, the practice of deceit and intellectual justification of actions that lead to evil.

Knowledge is a blessing for which thankfulness is expressed through guidance towards righteous actions, and the propagation and proclamation of these to those who are worthy. Ingratitude is the use of knowledge as an instrument of the passions, vainglory, causing dispute, and instructing the unworthy. Whoever gives knowledge to the unworthy wastes it and whoever withholds it from the worthy is an oppressor. This applies to all the limbs and faculties. So whenever they are aware of these blessings and the appropriate form of thankfulness for each one, they have attained thankfulness in knowledge which is the initial stage of thankfulness. When they have put this into practice, they will have attained thankfulness in practice which is the final stage. Thankfulness in knowledge is commonly expressed because of its simplicity, whereas thankfulness in practice is rare because of its excellence. The Quran states, "*Give thanks, oh family of David! Few of My devotees are thankful.*" (34:13)

STAGE 4
VIGILANCE

Being vigilant *(raqīb)* makes spiritual warriors aware of the fact that God sees them even if they do not see God. Recognizing this, the knowledge that God is aware of whatever is in their hearts as well as everything that they do brings about the positive disposition of vigilance according to Algazel whereby they are more watchful of their 'self' to act in accordance with God's Will manifest through nature's mode of operation. They seek the attention of the Responder to Prayer (al-Mujīb), so that the response is the Loving (al-Wadūd) as they continue to bear witness (*shāhid*) to the beauty and majesty of the Signs within and without. They develop a sense of peace or serenity as the verse, "*Oh self at peace, return to your Lord, well-pleased, well-pleasing,*" (89:27-28) seems to speak to spiritual warriors because they have continued to remember God and to invoke God following the verse, "*Be aware that only through remembrance of God may hearts become serene*" (13:28).

STAGE 5
TRUST

Spiritual warriors entrust themselves to God in this the sixth stage of moving towards perfection of the self. They manifest their portion of the Trustee (al-Wakīl) and the Friend (al-Walī) of God with humility and a sense of humbleness. They are no longer concerned with their false self but occupied with their duties. They begin to assume responsibility on their own behalf and are directed towards understanding responsibility on God's behalf.

Signs of their trust in God are not asking for things from others, not accepting things from others, and giving away whatever they have received from others. It means shedding their own power. According to the Quran, "*And trust in the Living Who never dies*" (25:58). Trust means abandoning volition or control, being liberated from their power. Once spiritual warriors become convinced that God is the doer and that God has complete knowledge and power and control over them as well as absolute mercy and providence, they develop a sincere trust in God and it is through this trust that they become the trustees of nature and the universe striving to maintain a balance and harmony by beginning with their own character healing.

Humility arises out of this. The humble person according to Algazel is "the one who intentionally gives up some of what he desires and in this way, implies self-abasement."[19] Realizing their true position in the universe, spiritual warriors can only become humble.

STAGE 6
REPENTANCE

Spiritual warriors then become a repenter (*tawwāb*), an avenger (*muntaqim*) of their heart and a pardoner (*'afū*) of their wrongdoings. Building on the resolve that spiritual warriors had strengthened in moving towards temperance, they consciously repent of worldly, personal desire and commit their 'self' to service of God and God's creation. They abandon everything which does not reinforce this within. They need to reproach their false self whenever it interferes with their goal by being an avenger (*muntaqim*) of the heart but to preserve moderation. They are also a pardoner (*'afū*) of the false self so that no guilt can cloud their healing.

Repentance means consciousness of the harm caused to the heart by wrongdoings. These wrongdoings veil spiritual warriors from all that they love. If their consciousness of this is accompanied by certitude, if their heart becomes convinced of this, a compassion arises in their 'self'. They sense pain for the separation they have from the heart. This pain is called remorse. When they are conscious of this pain, they resolve to act. Remorse, then, is the process or positive disposition and repentance is the product.

Repentance is to look to the past in terms of renouncing wrongdoing and to the present and future in terms of conflict resolution in order to heal. Repentance is a continuous obligation having its basis in the eternal tension between specific positive and negative traits. In the traditional view there is no universal negative trait like original sin. The self is born pure and it is nurture which turns it away from its original positive nature.

Repentance is to refrain from wrongdoing to the true self. Wrongdoing in the traditional perspective includes anything which distorts the relation between the self and its Divine Origin. The ultimate aim of the Law, in the view of psychoethics, is to guide spiritual warriors to their Divine Origin, the spiritual side of self. This can only come through knowing the spiritual origin of self which in turn leads them to the conclusion that they did not create their 'self' much less each other and therefore there must be a Creator Who sent guides to guide them to the Source. Since this awareness or consciousness can only come in this life, preservation of life and consciousness of the Source are essential to grow closer to their Source. Whatever obstructs spiritual warriors from consciousness of the Source is considered to be infidelity, the gravest of wrongdoing, followed by anything which shortens their life or deprives them of what they need to preserve their life in order to gain further consciousness. Once they realize that these wrongdoings of theirs separate and veil them from their Source, they reflect on each and every one of them, moment by moment, and turn away from or repent of those which distance them from their Source.

According to Algazel, if spiritual warriors have neglected a duty, they should discharge it. If they have done wrong to their Source, they should seek pardon. If they have wronged even a single creature, they should atone for it. If they have injured another they should comfort that person and make up for his or her suffering at their hands. If they have deprived someone of their possessions, they should restore them and seek the person's forgiveness.

Atonement can be made through the heart, speech or body. That done through their heart is the core of repentance. They achieve it by being a repenter (*tawwāb*) and seeking pardon from the Forgiver (al-Ghaffār), the Concealer of Faults (al-Ghafūr), the Pardoner (al-'Afū). Through speech they atone by acknowledging their wrongdoing and reciting a prayer for forgiveness. They physically atone through performing good deeds and prayer or fasting or giving to the poor.

The most difficult repentance to effect is repentance of the heart from errant thoughts and anxiety. It is effected by service to others, moving from seeking to avoid pain for the 'self' to helping others avoid pain and accompanies spiritual warriors for their entire lifetime.

Even if they free themselves from the wrongdoings of the body, they will still be anxious for them. Even if they free their 'self' from this anxiety, they will still fall short in remembrance of God; even if they are free of any shortcoming here, they will still be inadequate in their consciousness of God, God's Attributes and Acts. In order to effect the latter, they need both consciousness and patience, the next stage and last towards courage. Consciousness is the best way of guarding against the rebellion of their false self trying to postpone their perfecting self. Patience helps them resist the false self's pleas to do wrong or adopt the negative, it is necessary to reach the highest level of repentance which is that of the heart.

STAGE 7
PATIENCE

As spiritual warriors have become clement (*ra'ūf*) towards themselves, enricher (*mughnī*) of the potential of 'self', they are able to effect their inner guide (*hādī*). This is because they have become the patient (*ṣabur*) in regulating their avoidance of harm/pain.

Their consciousness of the need for patience (the process or positive disposition) produces action. The effect of the process is to remain patient and steadfast upon the Straight Path. The Messenger said, "... *Surah Hud* made an old man of me when it commanded me to remain steadfast..."

The lowest kind of patience is that of physical pain. The highest is the resistance to the demands of the passions. Spiritual warriors need patience at every stage of their life because they find their 'self' in basically two situations: either situations natural to them like health, safety, wealth and honor which when they confront with patience, they are safe from over indulging in them. Secondly, they may find themselves in situations which oppose their nature. These situations can be of three types: 1) they have to choose between following God's Will as it moves through nature's mode of operation or the will of their false self. Patience helps them follow God's Will; 2) a situation to which they have to react and can do so positively or negatively. For example if they have been wronged by another they may be able to resist revenge with patience; 3) situations completely out of their control like the death of a loved one or loss of health or wealth. Patience if manifest at this point instead of an outburst of passion, allows the true self to respond with satisfaction with God's decree.

There are two categories of patience: that which can be acquired and that which cannot be acquired. Patience which can be acquired is itself of two kinds: patience with what God has commanded and patience with what He has prohibited. As for that which cannot be acquired by the devotee, it is patience in enduring God's commands and resisting anger despite the suffering he or she may experience. "*So practice patience and your patience is through God alone*" (16:127).

According to Algazel, patience is one of the highest qualities possessed by mankind. It is not possessed by animals for they are dominated by the passions and do not have an intellect with which to combat them. Patience cannot be conceived of with respect to the angels either for they have a detached yearning for God, not being ruled by the passions such that they would be distracted from yearning for God and desire for nearness to Him. On the other hand, both the passions and the intellect exist in the human being, clashing with one another. Whenever the intellect succeeds in blocking the path of the passions, this is known as patience.

Chapter Three

Moral Healing of the Cognitive Function of the self Through Acquiring Wisdom

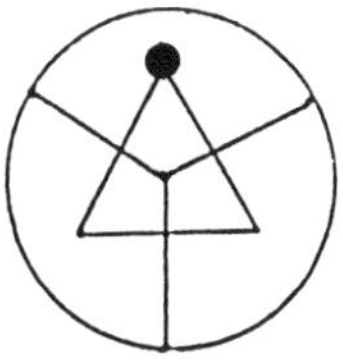

Wisdom develops from the cognitive faculty and it is of two types: theoretical and practical, both of which are called "intellect." The theoretical intellect is where spiritual warriors gather the imprints from external and internal sources which have to do with intelligible knowledge, in particular, that of the 'self' and of the Creator gained through observation or experience. If a person does not know the Creator, he or she may have completed the possibilities of the theoretical intellect, but not perfected it. The practical intellect is concerned with action and is the governor (*wālī*) or sovereign (*mālik*) over the self—and all physical, sensory, and psychical functions. The intellect is completed and perfected when it is processed through consciousness drawing on both aspects of the theoretical and the practical.

It can be said that the heart is purified, leading to the product of wisdom, when consciousness is the control tower for their attraction to pleasure—avoidance of harm as well as their cognition. This consciousness—as completing and perfecting God's Will in nature—leads spiritual warriors to being healed, centered in justice.

Wisdom is defined by Algazel as "a state and a virtue of the cognitive faculty which governs the attraction to pleasure and avoidance of harm faculty and it consists of positive actions"[1] and "a state of the self by which it perceives positive from negative in all voluntary actions"[2] and according to Naraqī, it is defined by the verse, "*who believe in God and then doubt not...*" (49:15)[3]

Consciousness, a state characterized by sensation, emotion, volition, and thought is considered to be rational, containing reason, when it engages in deliberation and is

Wisdom

Regulating the Cognitive Function Through Reason

Preserving the Eternal Possibility of Self

Cogniton

Learn to Think Differently

"Know yourself"

***"Believers are those who believe in God and His Messenger and then doubt not..."* (49:15)**

able to then choose the positive over the negative. It is to move out of unconsciousness (a state of depravity in terms of the quality of wisdom) and then effect moderation between overconsciousness or hypocrisy and preconsciousenss or multitheism. Overconsciousness is allowing the attraction to pleasure and avoidance of harm/pain faculties to move towards their desired object or action in a way which exceeds what is necessary. Preconsciousness is a state of the self which hinders the attraction to pleasure and avoidance of pain to reach the necessary amount.[4]

Avicenna and Ibn Miskawayh support this view of Algazel. Avicenna says, "By wisdom as a positive disposition, which is the third of a triad comprising in addition temperance and courage, is not meant theoretical wisdom—for moderation is not demanded in the latter at all—but, rather, practical wisdom pertaining to worldly actions and behavior. For it is deception to concentrate on the knowledge of this wisdom, carefully guarding the ingenious ways whereby one can attain through it every benefit and avoid every harm."[5]

The seven stages spiritual warriors move through in attaining wisdom or certitude in the belief in the One God are:

Stage 1: Aspiration
- al-Malik: The Sovereign
- al-Quddūs: The Holy
- al-Salām: The Flawless
- al-'Azīz: The Incomparable
- al-Mutakabbir: The Proud
- al-Qahhār: The Subduer

Stage 2: Self-Examination/Consciousness
- al-'Alīm: The Knower
- al-Samī': The All-Hearing
- al-Baṣīr: The All-Seeing
- al-Ḥakam: The Arbiter
- al-'Adl: The Just
- al-Laṭīf: The Subtle
- al-Khabīr: The Aware

Stage 3: Truthfulness
- al-'Aẓīm: The Magnificent
- al-'Alī: The Highest
- al-Kabīr: The Great
- al-Jalīl: The Majestic
- al-Karīm: The Generous
- al-Wāsi": The Vast
- al-Ḥakīm: The Wise
- al-Mājid: The Glorious
- al-Ḥaqq: The Truth

Stage 4: Contentment
- al-Qawī: The Strong
- al-Matīn: The Firm
- al-Ḥamīd: The Praised
- al-Ḥayy: The Living
- al-Qayyūm: The Self-Existing
- al-Wājid: The Resourceful
- al-Mājid: The Noble

Stage 5: Unity/Constancy
- al-Wāḥid: The Unique
- al-Aḥad: The One
- al-Ṣamad: The Eternal
- al-Qādir: The Able

Stage 6: Sincerity
- al-Awwal: The First
- al-Ākhir: The Last
- al-Ẓāhir: The Manifest
- al-Bāṭin: The Hidden

Stage 7: Remembrance
- al-Muta'ālī: The Exalted
- al-Barr: The Source of All Goodness
- Dhu 'l-Jalāl wa'l-Ikrām: The Lord of Majesty and Generosity
- al-Ghanī: The Rich
- al-Nūr: The Light
- al-Badī': The Originator
- al-Bāqī: The Everlasting

STAGE 1
ASPIRATION

Spiritual warriors aspire to heal their spiritual self or heart with which they were created. In order to do this, they must relinquish their inappropriate desires which may manifest themselves in terms of desires for food, sex, or material things or inappropriate anger. Aspiration means "attention of the heart on God with firm resolve towards attainment of perfection..."[6] which allows spiritual warriors to be a sovereign (*mālik*) over the self.

The Quran says, "*The eye [of the Messenger] did not wonder nor was overbold*" (53:17). Anṣārī says, "Aspiration is when one's sole control is in keeping one's motivation directed towards the object. The one who aspires has not control over himself and sees nothing other than aspiration."[7]

There are three degrees of aspiration according to another Sufi. "The first degree keeps one's heart from material desires that are transitory so that the heart concentrates on what is eternal (*ṣamad*) and holy (*quddūs*), cleansing the heart of the darkness of that which is transitory. The second degree engenders disregard for secondary causes, for the expectation of results from actions and for attachment to desires. The third degree is higher than states and stations because it uproots any thought of reward or degree..."[8]

And "... aspiration through God constitutes the tidings of success. It frees one from all other needs by focusing on a single need. It liberates one from all other attachments by fixing one on a single attachment and causes one to abandon all doors save entry through one particular door. One's aspiration is measured by one's value. That value has been His sign since pre-eternity and will be His seal until past-eternity."[9] It has been said in attaining a sense of the Holy (al-Quddūs): "...one who possesses aspiration is one who thinks of nothing without envisioning God."[10]

As Aṭṭār says, "Do not look at my lowly nature; look at

my aspiration."[11] Succeeding in relinquishing their flaws in their attempt to become flawless (*salām*) and being incomparable (*'azīz*) depends on the nature of their aspiration.

The worth of each person may be evaluated by the nature of his aspiration. If he aspires to worldly things, he is worthless. If he aspires to fulfill God's Will, it is impossible to assess, to comprehend, the extent of his worth."[12]

Through aspiration spiritual warriors differ from being a desirer of something which when attained makes them develop a false sense of being proud (*mutakabbir*). A distinction between aspiring with their heart and desires of their false self is made by a healer who said, "However deviant the one who aspires may be, he is close to soundness, whereas however correct the one who desires may be, he is a hypocrite. That is to say that the one who aspires does not desire an object such that he deviates from it at the slightest provocation. The reason is that one who aspires is not motivated by his own will power while the one who desires is easily satisfied and fickle."[13] Another said, "Be noble in aspiration for it is through noble aspiration that one attains the station of being a human being and not through mere striving."[14]

It is through aspiration that spiritual warriors become a subduer (*qahhār*) of their false self. "The aspiration of the great ones involves disregarding the false self (*nafs*) or ego which is the greatest evil that stands between you and God."[15]

They aspire to heal the self by allowing their consciousness to be the ruler (*malik*) of the self, healing their heart—which is the sacred and holy (*quddūs*) aspect of self. Through their aspiration they unveil the sacred aspect of self or heart, seeking to remove their flaws as they move towards being flawless, as they move towards healing their incomparable (*'azīz*) heart, allowing God to be the Proud (al-Mutakkabir).

STAGE 2
SELF-EXAMINATION

After performing some act, spiritual warriors reflect on it to see how close it is to what they had originally set as their goal—healing the self and how much they strayed from that goal. This is the stage of self-examination. If they find they have strayed from their goal and they are moving towards the false self instead of moving towards healing by purifying their heart, they should immediately reproach the self using their cognitive function. Their reproach should be appropriate (within moderation) to their wrongdoing.

If, on the other hand, their self-examination shows that they did not stray from their goal through any negative act but that they were lax in their commitment to the positive, then they have to will themselves to do more positive acts. If this proves to be too difficult, they can seek out believers and accompany them for awhile to reinstate the goal or read about believers and their experiences.

The final step in self-examination is to continue to reproach their tendencies towards inappropriate desires or anger. This is to strengthen their penetration of thought.

The following Quranic passage explicitly describes self-examination: "*Oh you who believe, be aware of God and look well into yourselves to see what you have in stock for tomorrow.*" (59:18). Through self-examination they seek to be a knower (*'alīm*) of their heart.

Those who truly practice self-examination possess certain characteristics which become manifested in their speech and action as aspects of their portion of the All-Hearing (al-Samī') and the All-Seeing (al-Baṣīr). This can take place, however, only by having a strong will and rejecting the inappropriate desires of the self. For one who acquires a strong will, opposition to the desires of the self will be easy. Thus it is essential to develop their will and to nurture the following characteristics which are known to bear fruit:

* Never swearing in the Name of God whether accidentally or deliberately, rightly or wrongly.

* Never lying.

* Never breaking a promise if at all feasible while avoiding making promises as much as possible.

* Never cursing another person (asking God to bring calamity upon that person) even one who has done harm.

* Never intending ill towards other people (whether in word or deed) or praying of them to be punished but rather tolerating everyone and everything for the sake of God.

* Never accusing another person of infidelity, multitheism, or the causing of discord—for accusing anyone of such acts is farther from having grace upon people and closer to the Divine wrath than refraining from such accusations.[16]

As an arbiter (*ḥakam*) of the self, in the words of the Messenger, "Take account of your actions before God takes account of you; weigh yourself before you are weighed; die before you die."

Algazel describes the best time for self-examination which is done by the self through a fair and just (*'adl*) accounting: "Just before going to sleep each night, the healer of the self should take account of what his self has done during the day so that his profits and losses get separated from his investments. The investments here are the necessary actions. The profits are the recommended actions and the losses are those actions which have been prohibited. Just as they would be cautious in buying something from a clever merchant, so they must bargain with caution in dealing with the self for the self is very tricky. It has a way of presenting its purposes in the garb of spiritual obedience so that they consider as profit what is really loss. In fact, in every action which is questionable, they should examine their motivation carefully. If it is determined that the motivation came from the self, then compensation should be demanded of it."[17]

Knowing the subtle (*laṭīf*) aspects of how they relate to

self and others is also important. Aṭṭār says that self-examination is:

* Never having the intention to commit wrongdoings either outwardly or inwardly (that is, dissociating one's whole being from everything that is not God).

* Never putting the burden of one's pain or suffering on anyone else's shoulders whether or not one's personal need is involved.

* Never having any greed whatsoever for any of the creations nor envying the possessions of others.

* Never considering oneself higher than any other human being—for in this way one will arrive at nearness to God both in this world and the world hereafter thereby attaining a high spiritual station and the perfection of honor.[18]

Through the manifestation of their portion of al-'Alīm (the Knower), al-Samī' (the All-Hearing), al-Baṣīr (the All-Seeing), al-Ḥakam (the Arbiter), al-'Adl (the Just) and al-Laṭīf (the Subtle) at the stage of self-examination, spiritual warriors gain consciousness and become aware (*khabīr*) of their heart and false self through their actions.

STAGE 3
TRUTHFULNESS

Cultivating their sense of the magnificent (*'aẓīm*) aspect of self as God's preferred creature who formed the covenant with God and accepted the trust, spiritual warriors keep their words consistent with their actions. They are able to become detached from the world as they rise above it (*'alī*), renouncing the seeking of the gratification offered by the world. They recognize that their healing lies in perfecting their inner greatness (*kabīr*), subduing the inappropriate desires and anger as they gain spiritual power (*jalīl*), not attempting to control things with the will of their false self. The vast (*wāsi'*) experience of the positive within us leads us to being wise (*ḥakīm*), doing what they say, possessing what they show to possess, and being what they claim to be. They perform good deeds (*majīd*) not allowing any temptation to violate their promises and expressing the truth (*ḥaqq*), being in accord with reality.

"Truthfulness can appear in six ways: through speech, intention, resolution, executing a resolution, action, and in attaining the various stages of temperance, courage, and wisdom. In speech it means to say something which is not only true but is unequivocal—not subject to be interpreted in various ways. In other words, it is to be honest with their true self when they engage in self-talk. It is to be honest with God when conversing with God as in prayer or spiritual monologue. They should say nothing that does not express their true spiritual state at that moment.

"Truthfulness of intention is to have only one aim for doing things and that is to draw closer to God. As regards resolution, it is to have the intention to do something when the circumstances arise to make it possible. Once this happens, they act without hesitation and with full power as truthfulness in execution of resolution. Truthfulness in action is when their inward state corresponds exactly to their outward acts without any indication of hypocrisy. The highest form of truthfulness is to fully and completely realize all of the stages towards healing the self. It is attained through clarity of mind when the self realizes it has the aptitude to obtain its goal without being waylaid by any agitation or confusion.

"The meaning of truthfulness is to stand watch over the self by guarding and observing it but first they must have fulfilled what is incumbent upon us according to the doctrine by setting up the proper bounds of outward states and having the right intention toward God at the outset of the act. Hence truthfulness is found within the reality of the attributes of will when the will undertakes to perform those things to which God has directed us and to which they are called by their will's reality. To accomplish this they refuse to conform to the self when it seeks ease, since the doctrine has been drawn up for us and they conform to it and they refuse to interpret the texts on their own.

"Hence truthfulness exists before the reality of sincerity. The Quran says, '*That He might question the truthful concerning their truthfulness*' (33:8). So He asked them what they wanted by their truthfulness after they had come to possess truthfulness. In another place, the Quran refers to the truthful in a different sense: '*This is the day the truthful shall be profited by their truthfulness.*' (5:119)

"Truthfulness is applied to three cases: the person who is truthful with his tongue and who speaks the truth, whether or not it be to his advantage, by leaving aside interpretation and falsification; the person who is truthful in his acts and who strives to the utmost to dislodge himself from ease; and the person who is truthful in his heart and who has the intention to go toward God through his acts. When a person possesses these traits he is truthful though truthfulness exists in the truthful person in every state. He is not free from it in any one of his states."[19]

STAGE 4
CONTENTMENT

Contentment is to be satisfied with whatever God Wills after striving. If their striving towards healing the self results in pain and hardship, spiritual warriors are content, strong (*qawī*) and firm (*matīn*) in having done their duty leaving the rest up to the Praiseworthy (al-Hamīd). Living (*ḥayy*) through the pain they take upon the self, detaching themselves (*qayyūm*) from everything but their goal, they become resourceful (*wajīd*) in finding what God wants us to find (*mājid*) when they have contentment.

With consciousness of their goal, the process of contentment, they delight in submitting to God's Will. This has now become their will, the perfecting of which is to attain consciousness of self for the Messenger said, "He who knows himself knows his Lord."

Healing masters have said: "Contentment is not a matter of being aware of affliction; contentment means not objecting to God's Will."[20] "Contentment with God for a devotee consists in setting aside his own volition before God's Will and being content with whatever God Wills, whether pleasant or unpleasant."[21] and "Contentment is the putting aside of free will."[22]

STAGE 5
UNITY/CONSTANCY

Unity means consciousness of the fact that God is One. Moral healers may do this in different ways—professing the unity of God with their lips but having no faith in their hearts or believing on the basis of authority like the majority of those who submit to the Will of God. The best way according to spiritual chivalry is to believe through their own deliberation for then they develop constancy.

Manifesting their aspects of being unique (*wāḥid*) and one (*aḥad*) they have died to their false self and now see and know nothing but God. "To consider oneself as oneself, as a separate entity, is to see God as two."[23]

Further deliberation on the One (al-Aḥad) leads to knowledge of the Eternal (al-Ṣamad).

* One who professes unity must distinguish between eternality and temporality; that is, he must know that with respect to the Essence, Attributes, and Acts, the Eternal is unlike the temporal.

* He must know that the temporal cannot attain the Eternal.

* He must not consider God's Attributes equal to those of created beings.

* He must know that God is too great to be affected of His view altered by the power of the temporal. In other words, His pleasure is not earned by obedience nor His anger by disobedience. Service is not rewarded by proximity nor does infidelity lead to distance. If the opposite were true, the Eternal would have to be considered as mutable would be absurd."[24]

Once they have recognized the Eternal (al-Ṣamad) aspect of the One (al-Aḥad), the Unique (al-Waḥīd), they are able (*qādir*) to cut their self from all with which their false self is familiar in the process healing their self.

Unity of self "is to make the heart one, that is, to purify it and disengage it from attachment to anything other than God both in terms of aspiration and desire and in terms of theory and knowledge. In other words, the aspiration and desire are cut off from all objects and all objects of knowledge, all intelligible things, are removed from the eye of his insight. He turns his attention away from every other direction so that his consciousness and awareness remain fixed upon none but God."[25]

In terms of constancy, this means following the verse, "*Be constant towards Him*!" (41:6). Constancy of moral traits has three signs: If people are cruel toward you, you ask their pardon; if they torment you, you give thanks; and if they become sick, you go to visit them. Constancy of breathes has three witnesses: you watch over each breath, in order to gain worth; you consider your lifetime a single breath in order to become free; and you scrutinize the breath in order to become fulfilled. Know that at each passing breath your life is either a disputant or an intercessor. With each breath God shows kindness to the servant while in face of that the servant commits wrongdoing. A miserable breath is the smoke of a snuffed out lamp in a narrow, doorless room, while a fortunate breath is a radiant fountain in a garden adorned with fruit.[26]

They manifest constancy as they become a model that is eternal (*ṣamad*) for humankind, empowered as they are and able (*qādir*) from having further perfected their consciousness and will power.

STAGE 6
SINCERITY

Sincerity is when spiritual warriors act with one intention alone in mind. This is single-mindedness in purpose and the positive trait applies in psychoethics and healing the self when they have one intention and that is to heal their self without any selfish or worldly intention or motive. Attaining sincerity means they have overcome or gone beyond the reach of their false self or ego. The Quran says, "Satan said, '*Then by Your power I will deceive them all save Your sincere servants among them*'" (38:82-83).

Sincerity is manifested when they have one basic resolve or intention behind their actions. If other intentions are mixed in—for instance, fasting to lose weight, they have not attained this stage. Their sole intention needs to be closeness to God in order to be able to effect sincerity.

This they know through discernment towards the "mothers of the character traits"—the First (al-Awwal), the Last (al-Ākhir), the Manifest (al-Ẓahir) and the Hidden (al-Baṭīn). "The first (*awwal*) step is sincerity is to devote oneself exclusively to God through the will." "*Assuredly They purified them with a quality of sincerity*." (38:46).[27] "It has been said sincerity is that you seek no witness for your actions but God."[28]

"Sincerity is when man's outward and his inward, his stillness and his movement, are purely for God, not stained by gratification of the self, passion, creation, or desire."[29]

"What thing is hardest for the self? Sincerity since the self has no share in it."[30] "When you do something while seeking God, that is sincerity, but when you do something while seeking the creatures, that is hypocrisy. What need is there in the midst for creatures? God is the place for sincerity."[31] "Sincerity is God's goal for the creatures in which He has called them to worship."[32]

STAGE 7
REMEMBRANCE

Reflection (*fikr*) is "bringing together two ideas in order to produce from them a third one." [33] Spiritual warriors have brought knowledge and action together by expressing the healing process. The Messenger said, "An hour's meditation is more excellent than a year's worship."[34]

When their healing process is oriented towards carrying out the trust which has been given them, spiritual warriors use reflection to better understand their self, their relations to others, and their relations to their Source, the Exalted (al-Muta'ālī), the Source of All Goodness (al-Barr), the Lord of Majesty and Generosity (Dhū 'l-Jalāl wa 'l-Ikrām). Through reflection their inner meaning becomes rich (*ghani*) and full of the light (*nūr*) of insight. They have succeeded in being an originator (*badī'*) of their recreated self by this time consciously participation in the process through the exercise of their own free-will and conscience. They have freely chosen to recreate their self in God's image as they were originally created and they have placed an emphasis on that part of self which is everlasting (*bāqī*).

The most important kind of meditation and reflection according to Algazel is when spiritual warriors reflect upon their character traits and actions towards others based as they are now in knowledge of the operations of God's Trust given to them as trustees (theoethics) to the extent humanly possible.

At this stage of moral growth, they know the self is divided into a heart given to them by nature and a false self or ego assumed little by little through the nurturing process. Both of these have external and internal qualities, the actions of their heart relate to their inner meaning (psychoethics) and their relations with others (socioethics). The same is true of their false self. Each of these, in turn, can be positive leading to their attaining the highest level—being a human being in the full sense of the word or the negative being a product of their own creation because they further the nurturing process instead of emphasizing their natural state. "This leads us to reflect on God's mysterious and wonderful works manifested in the creations because all of these show God's glory, majesty, knowledge, and power."[35] "Meditation is the means through which the self performs its 'natural' role of reflecting on the highest truth."[36] Since this can only be expected of a self which has subjugated its lower faculties [to reason], meditation is among the highest levels of positive traits.

Chapter Four

Centering The Self with Justice

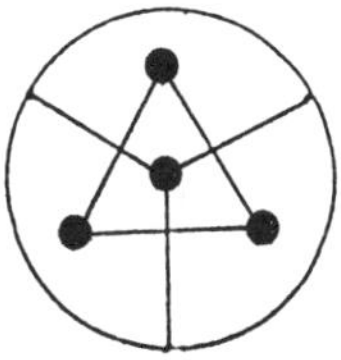

Having left aside all negative traits of the various faculties, spiritual warriors begin to heal the true self by denouncing, reproaching, and diminishing the importance of the false self or ego. Of their three major faculties of self—affect, behavior and cognition, they begin with affect. They move through seven stages of perfecting their motivations through which God disclosed Self in creation—assuming their portion of the Most Beautiful Names that related to each stage at each level in order to move from the most material aspect of their instinctive nature—attraction to pleasure/affect—to the highest state it can attain, that of temperance and self-restraint.

Justice

Being centered in wisdom, temperance and courage.

Balanced

***"Believers are those who believe in God and His Messenger and then doubt not, and strive with their wealth in the Way of God and strive with their lives in the Way of God; they are the truthful ones."* (49:15)**

They then turn towards perfecting their instinct of avoidance of harm/behavior by transforming it through their perceptions into courage where they put their 'self' in risk-taking situations in order to serve all creatures but particularly their fellow human beings. Again, they move through seven stages, perfecting their portion of each of the Most Beautiful Names that God disclosed for humanity.

Finally, perfecting their motivations, the highest form of which is free will and their perceptions, the highest form of which is conscience, through seven stages, they gained an understanding of the Most Beautiful Names through which God disclosed Self.

Their true 'self' then is self-restraining, patient, and a rememberer. It is then that the self—if fully healed—will manifest justice if another person benefits from the healed self. If they have healed, they now manifest justice. It has been defined traditionally as Plato defined it, "When the faculty of justice develops in the human being, all other faculties and powers of the self are illuminated by it and these faculties and powers acquire light from each other. This is the condition in which the human self moves and acts in the best and the most meritorious manner possible, gaining affinity and rapprochement with the Source of creation."[1]

In terms of process, being centered in justice saves spiritual warriors from the danger of extremes in both personal and social issues. Until they do not find centeredness, they cannot be just and fair towards others in society. If each individual heals the self, then society will also be healed or that community in which the healed reside will be a healed community, balanced and centered just as nature is centered in harmony and unity.

Part III: The Actions of Spiritual Warriors: Proof of Moral Healing Through Socioethics

"We all show them Our Signs upon the horizons...until it is clear to them that it is the Real (the Truth)" (41:53)

Part I gives spiritual warriors the knowledge of how the Absolute Self-discloses through the Most Beautiful Names. They become the norm for them to the extent humanly possible to attain. In other words, assuming the Most Beautiful Names depends upon the receptivity of the spiritual warrior. Part II developed the process of this knowledge and how it works through individually assuming a portion of the Most Beautiful Names in moving from inappropriate desires to moderation, balance and temperance; through inappropriate anger to moderation, balance and courage; through reason and consciousness of God, wisdom in the view of spiritual chivalry, and total self balance and moderation. When all three positive traits—expressions of God's Self-disclosure through the Most Beautiful Names to creation, to humanity, and in Self—are held in moderation with control in reason, spiritual warriors attain to the fourth positive trait of justice but only if another person verifies this for them. Part III tests the results of the endeavors of spiritual warriors by relating to other people through the Most Beautiful Names. This part holds the action of the knowledge they have gained and the healing process they have experienced.

The major divisions of the Ninety-Nine Names in testing the relationships of spiritual warriors with others are ten. These divisions have been developed to further the learning process of understanding the Most Beautiful Names as manifested in the noble character traits. The proof of success in Parts I and II is the actions of spiritual warriors in their relationships as individuals with others. They come to understand the noble character traits as the most excellent guides to communication skills by incorporating the Most Beautiful Signs of God in the universe in their relations with others. As mentioned in the Preface, all illustrations and analogies are translated from Rūmī unless otherwise indicated.

The stations are:

Chapter 1: Social Awakening by Emptying the Heart of Everything But the Desire to Grow Closer to God

- al-Raḥmān: The Merciful
- al-Raḥīm: The Compassionate
- al-Malik: The Sovereign
- al-Quddus: The Holy
- al-Salām: The Flawless
- al-Mu'min: The Giver of Faith
- al-Muhyamin: The Guardian
- al-'Azīz: The Incomparable
- al-Jabbār: The Compeller
- al-Mutakabbir: The Proud

Chapter 2: Entering the Creative Process

- al-Khāliq: The Creator
- al-Bāri': The Maker of Perfect Harmony
- al-Muṣawwir: The Shaper of Unique Beauty
- al-Ghaffār: The Forgiver
- al-Qahhār: The Subduer
- al-Wahhāb: The Bestower
- al-Razzāq: The Provider
- al-Fattāḥ: The Opener
- al-'Alīm: The Knower

Chapter 3: Counseling to the Positive and Trying to Prevent the Development of the Negative

- al-Qābiḍ: The Constrictor
- al-Bāsiṭ: The Expander
- al-Khāfiḍ: The Abaser
- al-Rāfi': The Exalter
- al-Mu'izz: The Honorer
- al-Mudhill: The Dishonorer
- al-Samī': The All-Hearing
- al-Baṣīr: The All-Seeing
- al-Ḥakam: The Arbiter
- al-'Adl: The Just
- al-Laṭīf: The Subtle
- al-Khabīr: The Aware

Chapter 4: Developing the Moral Reasonableness of a Religiously Cultured Person

- al-Ḥalīm: The Forebearer

al-'Aẓim: The Magnificent
al-Ghafūr: The Concealer of Faults
al-Shakūr: The Rewarder of Thankfulness
al-'Alī: The Highest
al-Kabīr: The Great
al-Ḥafīẓ: The Preserver
al-Muqīt: The Maintainer
al-Ḥasīb: The Reckoner
Chapter 5: Using Their Spiritual Power to Help Others
al-Jalīl: The Majestic
al-Karīm: The Generous
al-Raqīb: The Vigilant
al-Mujīb: The Responder to Prayer
al-Wāsi': The Vast
al-Ḥakīm: The Wise
al-Wadūd: The Loving
al-Majīd: The Glorious
al-Bā'ith: The Resurrector
al-Shahīd: The Witness
al-Ḥaqq: The Truth
Chapter 6: Trusting in God
al-Wakīl: The Trustee
al-Qawī: The Strong
al-Matīn: The Firm
al-Walī: The Friend
al-Ḥamīd: The Praised
al-Muḥṣī: The Appraiser
al-Mubdi': The Beginner
al-Mu'īd: The Restorer
Chapter 7: Perfecting their Instinctive Perception Through Noble Character Development
al-Muḥyī: The Life-Giver
al-Mumīt: The Slayer
al-Ḥayy: The Living
al-Qayyūm: The Self-Existing
al-Wājid: The Resourceful
al-Mājid: The Noble
al-Wāḥid: The Unique
al-Aḥad: The One
al-Ṣamad: The Eternal

Chapter 8: Perfecting or Instinctive Motivation Through Noble Character Development

al-Qādir: The Able
al-Muqtadir: The Powerful
al-Muqaddim: The Promoter
al-Mu'akhkhir: The Postponer
al-Awwal: The First
al-Ākhir: The Last
al-Ẓāhir: The Manifest
al-Bāṭin: The Hidden
al-Wālī: The Governor
al-Muta'ālī: The Exalted
al-Barr: The Source of All Goodness
al-Tawwāb: The Acceptor of Repentance
al-Muntaqim: The Avenger
al-'Afū: The Pardoner

Chapter 9: Moving Towards Servanthood by Serving God's Creation

al-Ra'ūf: The Clement
Mālik al-Mulk: The King of Absolute Sovereignty
Dhū'l-Jalāl wa 'l-Ikrām: The Lord of Majesty and Generosity
al-Muqsit: The Equitable
al-Jāmi': The Gatherer
al-Ghanī: The Rich
al-Mughnī: The Enricher
al-Māni': The Protecter
al-Nāfi': The Punisher
al-Ḍārr: The Creator of the Beneficial

Chapter 10: Serving as a Guide and Teacher to Others

al-Nūr: The Light
al-Hādī: The Guide
al-Badī': The Originator
al-Bāqī: The Everlasting
al-Wārith: The Inheritor
al-Rashīd: The Right in Guidance
al-Ṣabur: The Patient

Chapter One

Social Awakening by Emptying the Self of Everything but the Desire to Grow Closer to God

Emptying their heart of love of their false self or ego, spiritual warriors begin to awaken to a new sense of their real self in their relations to others. They begin a paradigm shift by consciously, in full awareness of what they are doing, letting their mercy (*raḥamā*) precede their wrath. Having emptied their heart of everything but the desire to grow closer to God through serving God's people, they are compassionate (*raḥīm*) towards believers. They force their power of reason to predominate over any inappropriate anger or desires in their relations with others (*malik*). Cleansing their heart (*quddūs*) of any prejudgments and prejudices towards others, they concentrate on developing healthy, relatively flawless (*salām*) relationships by avoiding the negative. When they sense the pain of their loss of false self or tend to slip back into previous patterns of imbalance, disharmony, and chaos, they seek refuge in their faith (*mu'min*). They guard against wronging others (*muhaymin*), consciously striving to overcome the powers which may divide them from their friends (*'azīz*), implementing God's Will (*jabbār*) and crushing any egotism or pride (*mutakabbir*) that may remain during this stage of awakening.

Application

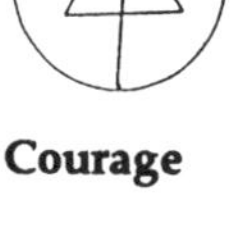

Courage

One sign of those who have courage is that they are merciful (*raḥmān*), make friends easily and do not force their own opinions on those around them. This quality of universal mercy may be actualized in adulthood through having had parents who understood and practiced the Divine Tradition (*ḥadith qudsī*), "My mercy precedes my wrath." Such parents do not coerce their children into following their belief system. They remind their children of their duties—duties which the parents themselves regularly practice—counsel them to the positive (*amr bi' l-ma' ruf*) and try to prevent the development of the negative (*nahy an al-munkar).* In every instance, the parents love for their children precedes their wrath or anger and they are gentle in their approach, looking upon their children if they fail in their obligations, with mercy and not disdain or anger. Over the years, their children come to realize that parents do this for the benefit of their children because each person alone will be responsible before God. Proof of mercy being reflected by parents is twofold: first of all, God blesses them with His mercy so that they sense the Will of His total goodness. In response, they chose to submit to His Will and to work for the good of others. Secondly, they are very sensitive towards the psychological pain and suffering felt by anyone who is misguided to which they respond with sympathy and whatever assistance they can offer.

In order for mercy to be universal, it should be extended towards all creatures, not just their own family. Their sense of mercy should include all of nature—inanimate and animate, believers and non-believers. It is a sign in us which responds to the heart in others, not their false ego. When they reflect this sign, they show no pride in their good deeds because they know that everything comes from God, including whatever it is they have.

There are many examples of mercy among human beings. Once a young man in his late teens was walking down a street in Lahore when suddenly he saw a man from the electric company fall from the top of an electric pole. Having heard the sound of electricity passing through an object and having seen the sparks, he realized the man was in shock from both having been electrocuted and falling. Without thinking or even realizing that he had no money with him, he hailed a taxi, picked the man up, and rushed him to the nearest hospital. Unfortunately the man was dead on arrival but the young man never forgot the experience of the pain and sympathy he felt nor of the speed with which mercy (*raḥamā*) can be made manifest. He became someone who pursued the course of spiritual chivalry.

Children learn the lesson of mercy from their parents which gives strength to their faith. Their strength of faith, in turn, creates a love in all those to whom they relate. In a Tradition reported by 'Alī, the Messenger responded to a question about "compassionate among themselves (the believers)," (48:29) saying, "The self which is dearest to God is firm in religion, pure in faith and kind toward believers."

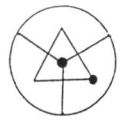

Courage

The same young man had been born into a large family. His six brothers and sisters attest to the fact that he was a merciful (*raḥmān*) person from a very early age. From the time he began going to school, he gave whatever money his parents gave him for food, to the poor sitting at his school entrance. He quickly placed the money in their hands and ran into the school yard hoping no one would ever know how kind hearted he was. What his family noticed was that not only was he merciful towards all creatures but showed courage in that he was compassionate (*raḥīm*) towards believers. The young man volunteered to help out at the local hospital where he concentrated his efforts on helping believers based on the verse, *"God is Compassionate towards the believers"* (33:43). When he went to the hospital, he saw that every patient there needed his attention. As he was the only volunteer, he had to become selective and he remembered this verse and performed good deeds because of his compassion for the believers.

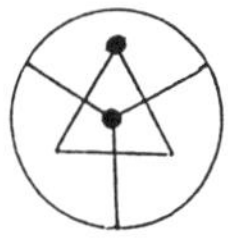

Wisdom

The need for the manifestation of sovereignty (*malik*) or rulership in a relationship is one of the most difficult Signs to bear, requiring wisdom. Once a prince asked a mystic to call upon him, the prince, for whatever it was that the mystic needed. The mystic said, "How can you possibly ask me that when I have two servants who are your masters?" The prince asked, "Who are these two?"

The mystic responded, "Inappropriate anger and desires. I have conquered them with reason while they have conquered you. I rule over them while they rule over you."

Another prince asked a shaykh to advise him how to proceed with his rule. The shaykh responded, "Be a king (*malik*) in this world, having wisdom and discernment, you will be a king in the next." The prince asked, "How can I do that?" The shaykh responded, "Detach yourself in this world from inappropriate anger and lust because kingship lies in being balanced."

The moral in terms of relationships is that when spiritual warriors can control their irrational parts of the self through reason, the self is then freed to reflect. From this reflection comes the certain belief that they are all totally dependent on God alone. Having disciplined the ego or false self (the animal within), they are able to form more healthy, long lasting relationships with others.

A thirsty man discovered a brick walled well but could not drink of it because it was surrounded by a high wall. He took some of the bricks off the top of the wall and threw them into the water. The water cried out, "What advantage do you gain by doing this?" He answered, "The more bricks I throw into the water from the wall, the nearer I approach to you." The moral is that so long as the wall of inappropriate desires and anger intervene, spiritual warriors cannot reach the water of life. The disciplining of them brings human beings closer to their spiritual side and further from their false self.

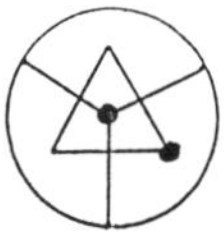

Courage

Continuing their efforts to lighten their hearts from the burdens of attachment to worldly things, manifesting wisdom, spiritual warriors cleanse their heart (*quddūs*) of pre-judgment of others. What happens so often is that people look only at outward form and then proceed to judge a person without regard to their spirit and essential self.

A wise man once told a king that there was a tree of such wonderful fruit in India that whoever ate of the tree lived forever. The king immediately sent one of his

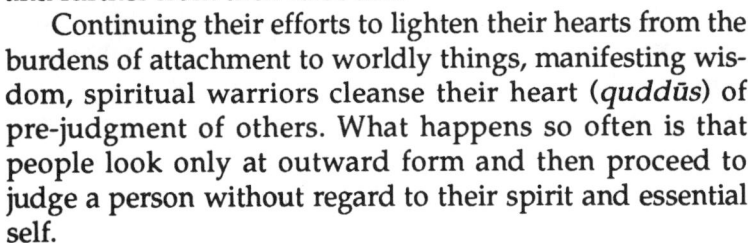

courtiers in search of the tree. He traveled throughout India in search of it asking anyone he saw where he could find this tree. Some persons professed ignorance, others joked with him, and others gave him false information. The courtier finally returned home with his mission unaccomplished and sought out the sage who had told the king of this tree, asking the mystic for more information.

The mystic replied that the courtier had been running after the form rather than spirit and that is why he had failed. He said, "I am referring to the tree of knowledge which is very high, very fine, very expansive, the water of life of the ocean. Sometimes it is named 'tree', sometimes 'sun', sometimes 'lake', and sometimes 'cloud'. It is one but has many manifestations, the least of which is eternal life. Its names are innumerable just as someone they meet may be a father to one and a son to another or mother to one and daughter to another. That person may act with anger and vengeance towards one person and with mercy and goodness towards another. The person may have many relational names yet is one, answering all descriptions yet being indescribable. If you seek after names," the mystic told the courtier, "you will remain hopeless and frustrated. Why do you cleave to the mere name of this tree? Pass over names and look to qualities so that qualities may lead you to essence." This includes not relating to others through cultural biases and stereotyping which serve to divide human beings from each other rather than to unify them.

Clearly when spiritual warriors relate to others to whom they are intimate only through their outward forms, they can be easily led into error and delusion. Once four people, a Persian, an Arab, a Turk, and a Greek were traveling together. Someone gave the four of them one dirham. The Persian said he would buy *angur*; the Arab said he would buy *inab*; while the Turk and Greek each said respectively that they would buy *uzum* and *astaphil*. Each of these four words means the same thing—grape—but because each was not familiar with the language of the other, they began to argue thinking each wanted to buy something different with the dirham that had been given to them. A wise man finally explained to them that they each wanted the same thing.

How does the spiritual warrior become a ruler of the self? Algazel draws the following analogies: The self is a sovereign (*malik*) over the body just as a king is sovereign over an empire. In the empire of the self, hands, feet and their other organs are like the citizens of the empire. Attraction to pleasure or desire is the tax collector and avoidance of harm or anger is as its police. Reason is the prime minister. As long as all the citizens including the tax collector and police are under the rule of reason, the empire is at peace and the self or sovereign is in control. The self at times seeks the help of reason to control desires, keeping anger in control and, at other times, to keep anger in control, it seeks the help of the tax collector. The Quran speaks about the self not controlled by reason, saying, "*Do you not see the one who takes for his deity his own desires?...*" (25:43) One who follows the attraction to pleasure function is like a dog— " *...if you attack it, it sticks out its tongue or if you leave it alone, it still sticks out its tongue...*" (7:176). On the other hand, in regard to those who follow their reason it says, "*And for such as had entertained the fear of standing before their Lord's (tribunal) and had restrained (their souls) from their desires*" (79:40).

Another example is to see their body as a town over which reason or conscience rules like a sovereign *(malik)*. The army consists of their internal and external senses and the subjects are their limbs and organs. Attraction to pleasure and avoidance of harm are the enemies of the town which reason guards against. If reason fights against its enemies and defeats them, the actions of the subjects become commendable. "*Those who believe and suffer exile and strive with their might in God's cause with their goods and their persons have the highest rank in the sight of God. They are the people who will achieve (salvation)*" (9:20).

Because as human beings, spiritual warriors are not

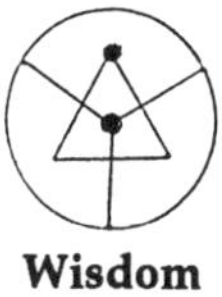

Wisdom

flawless (*salām*), it often happens in their relations with others that they notice their negative qualities as so many shadows of their own qualities with which they have yet to deal. They develop many negative traits from childhood. For instance, because of their cultural background, they may grow up in a home where they are taught never to say what they feel. They learn to hide their true feelings and develop hypocrisy towards others. They may tell their friend how good they think she looks while inside they say to themselves, "She really looks terrible. Yellow does not suit her at all." Or they may be jealous of their friends and envious towards anyone who has something they do not have. They have to blame themselves whenever any one of these traits appears. They may talk to the self as often as possible trying to understand why they have failed once again, forcing themselves to apologize to anyone they hurt. Often this apology will be accompanied by tears. They will begin to develop their sense of wisdom and contentment with what they have instead of desiring what others have.

They learn not to find fault with others, but rather to learn from their flaws and bad example. Once four Muslims went to the mosque to offer their afternoon prescribed prayer. Each one pronounced the *takbir al-ihrām*, forbidding anything but the prescribed prayer to follow. The Muslims were praying with great devotion when the person who calls out the prayer (*mu'adhdhin*) came into the mosque. In the middle of the prescribed prayer, one of them called out, "Have you called the people to the prescribed prayer? It is time to do so." Then the second said to the speaker, also interrupting his prescribed prayer, "So and so, you have spoken words unconnected with worship and therefore have invalidated your prayer." The third scolded the second, again, in the middle of his prayer, saying, "Why do you reproach him? Reproach yourself!" The fourth one then said, interrupting his prayer just as the others had done, "God be praised that I have not fallen into the same trap as my three companions."

Another story with similar moral is traditionally told where two prisoners were captured by a group of tribal warriors. The warriors were about to put one of the two prisoners to death in order to frighten the other and make him confess where he had buried the treasure they had stolen. When the doomed man realized what was happening, he said, "Oh noble tribesmen, kill my companion and frighten me instead!"

Little by little spiritual warriors realize that their reasoning powers, not rationalizing powers, have to stay in control and regulate their feelings and behavior. Whenever they forget to reason with themselves, one of their negative traits will surface. A hunter went out to catch birds and disguised himself by wrapping his head up in leaves and grass so as to avoid frightening the birds away from his snare. A bird of some wisdom came near him and suspected something was wrong but foolishly lingered near and began to question him as to his business. The hunter said he was a hermit who had retired from the world and dressed himself in weeds for the health of his soul. The bird said it was surprised to see a Muslim doing this in contravention of the Prophet's precept, "There is no monasticism in Islam," and his repeated declarations that Islam involves association with the faithful and avoidance of a solitary life. The hunter replied that a solitary life was allowed in heathen countries for the self's health. The bird then asked what the grains of wheat were that were strewed on the trap. The hunter replied that they were the property of an orphan which had been deposited with him in consequence of his trustworthiness. The bird then asked permission to eat some, as it was very hungry. The hunter, with much pretended reluctance, allowed it to do so. The moment it touched the grain, the trap closed upon it and it found itself a prisoner. It then abused the hunter for his tricks but the hunter said the bird had only itself to blame for its greediness in eating the food which belonged to an orphan.

Spiritual warriors learn that it is not destiny that leads

us astray, but their own errors and negative traits. To follow the sign of flawlessness they must free their heart of fraud, hatred, envy, and the desire for evil. They need to develop a spiritual healthiness in their relations towards others. Once their reason dominates over their negative traits of inappropriate desires and anger in their relationships with others, they become people from whose hand and tongue other believers are safe. Then they manifest a portion of the sign of justice, their portion of the Flawless (al-Salām).

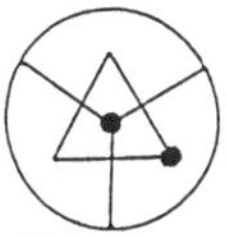

Courage

Lovers of God have heartaches for which neither sleep nor food proves to be of any avail. They seek refuge in the Giver of Faith (*al-Mu' min*) and help others to attain faith. In this way, it is as if they are meeting the Friend and the effects upon those who do not believe can be amazing as the Quran says, "*When they meet those who believe, they say, 'We believe'*." So much so, then, the effects of believers sitting with believers. Think about how wool, by just being near an intelligent person, becomes a beautiful, multi-designed carpet; how earth, being near an intelligent person, becomes a palace. When they see the effects of inanimate things on a society of intelligent people, consider the effect the company of a believer, who manifests courage, can have on another believer.

Those who move towards faithlessness join the non-believers. Those whose words and actions confirm a faith that is not in their hearts are deceiving themselves and others. They have developed hypocrisy and turned away from fidelity to the One God. Being a person whom others can depend upon and one who does not deny help to those in need are manifestations of the sign of the Giver of Faith (*al-Mu' min*).

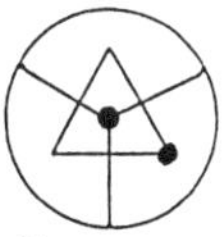

Courage

Guarding against wronging others (*muhaymin*), manifesting a sense of courage, requires consciousness of one's thoughts, words, and deeds. Protecting the rights of others or obtaining the rights others have lost is the other side of the quality of being a guardian.

When spiritual warriors are in command of the situation they are in, when they take control and protect it, they are manifesting the sign of a guardian (*muhaymin*). When they are in command of the situation, they have knowledge. When they take control, they have the perfection of power and when they are able to protect the situation, they are in action. In their relationships with others, when they try to help friends stay on the Straight Path after becoming aware of their inner states or inferring them from their behavior, spiritual warriors' portion of this quality is even greater.

At the same time, they follow the adage, "Don't make friends with fools." A kind man, seeing a snake about to kill a bear, went to the bear's rescue and saved him from the snake. The bear was so appreciative of the kindness the man had done him that it followed him about wherever he went and became his faithful slave, guarding him from everything that might annoy him. One day the man was lying asleep and the bear, according to its custom, was sitting by him and driving off the flies. The flies became so persistent in their annoyances that the bear lost patience. Seizing the largest stone it could find, it threw it at at the flies in order to crush them. Unfortunately the flies escaped but the stone landed on the sleeper's face and crushed it. The man, through establishing an incomparable relationship, forgot common sense.

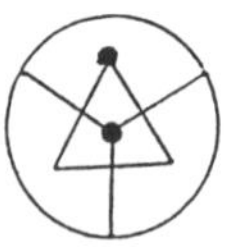
Wisdom

Seeking victory over the powers which divide spiritual warriors from their friends and controlling those powers in their relationships is a sign of their wisdom operative in their relationship allowing each and everyone to be incomparable (*'azīz*) to the other. With this quality they grow strong. This strength is such that they will not let themselves be divided from their friends

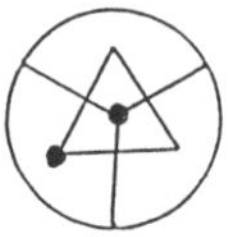
Temperance

They see God's Will at work in creation and learn that only by joining their will to His can they succeed in manifesting this quality, letting go of their false self and tempering its desires, they begin to submit to God's Will manifest through the Compeller (al-Jabbār). God 'speaks' words of power to the inner forces in nature—to inanimate things which have no eyes or ears, who spring into being with God's Command. God also 'speaks' to beings. God 'speaks' into the rose's 'ear' and causes it to bloom, 'speaks' to the tulip and it suddenly blossoms, 'speaks' to a body and it discovers 'self', 'speaks' to the sun and it becomes a fountain of light. Again, at another time, God whispers a word of power and the light of the sun is eclipsed by the moon. What does God say to the earth that it nourishes and gives forth? What does God say to a cloud that it gives forth the rain?

When it comes to human beings, the difference between God's actions and ours is clear. Rumi explains,

If the heart opens the mouth of mystery's store,
The self springs up swiftly to the highest heaven.
If the tongue discourses on hidden mysteries,
It kindles a fire that consumes the world.
Behold, then, God's action and human actions
Know, action does belong to us. This is evident.
If no actions proceeded from human beings,
How could you say, "Why can't you do this?" "or
    that?"
The agency of God is the cause of our action
Our actions are the Signs of God's agency
Nevertheless our actions are freely willed by us
Therefore our reward is either hell or 'The Friend'.

The purpose behind enforcing God's Will within the self for spiritual warriors and overcoming their own ego and its desires is to discipline their 'self'. God gave human beings free will to revolt against His Will but He also gave them the wisdom to know right from wrong. The goal of His Will within is to find God and to become God's servants (*'abid*). People are not made to do this. They are not forced to do this. They can choose to ignore this. But when they reflect on God's ability to compel all other creatures in nature to follow His Will, they realize that God is their refuge, as well. The Sign to them of the manifestation of al-Jabbar within them is their very reflection on It as the force which dominates everything. It is then that spiritual warriors also try to enforce God's Will and efface their own.

Little by little, manifesting wisdom, they will realize that any fame or position that they have attained or any knowledge they have gained is but momentarily theirs. That which is eternal belongs to God alone. At one point spiritual warriors realize that they had been no more than a sperm united with an egg in their mother's womb. They learn not to have a sense of arrogance in their accomplishments because they know that success comes from God alone. The quality *al-Mutakabbir,* the Proud, belongs to God in His greatness in comparison to their smallness. Those who fail at this stage, those who are still self-centered, egotistical, haughty, and arrogant towards others will be humiliated by this very same quality.

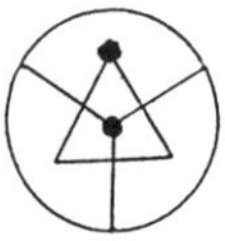

Wisdom

Fear not to acknowledge your ignorance and guilt
That the heavenly Master may not withhold instruction.
When you say, "I am ignorant, teach me,"
Such open confession is better than false pride.
O ingenuous one, learn of our father Adam
Who said, "O Lord, they have been unjust."
He made no vain excuses
Nor did he raise the standard of guile and cunning.

Chapter Two
Entering the Creative Process

To this point spiritual warriors have learned how the noble traits of awakening to the desire to draw closer to God are manifested in social relationships. In the second phase they will emphasize the creative process. The first three noble traits center around the concept of creativity. As noble character traits, spiritual warriors intend to create their relationships (*khāliq*) in perfect harmony (*bāri'*) in shapes of unique beauty (*muṣawwir*). Part of the creative process in transforming their relationships is to conceal the secrets of their friends, being reminded themselves that God is the Forgiver (*al-Ghaffār*). They find creative ways to strengthen their will power and that of their community (*ummah*) to overcome its enemies within and without (*qahhār*) and they give to others (*wahhāb*). Through the creative process, their relationships with others grow rich in spirituality (*razzāq*), as they seek out the keys to the secrets of knowledge (*fattāḥ*) and ask for an increase in intuitive wisdom (*'alīm*).

Application

The Creator (al-Khāliq), The Maker of Perfect Harmony (al-Bāri'), and the Shaper of Unique Beauty (al-Muṣawwir) refer to the process of creation. In terms of socioethics, it is to manifest temperance. To be a creator (*khāliq*) for spiritual warriors is to conceive of the possibilities of things for spiritual warriors, to develop their searching mind to go beyond what is obvious or superficial. Being among those who are trying to assume or take on the noble character traits, they conceive of the possibilities of them. Their creative striving is in response to "*God changes not what is in a people until they change what is in themselves*" (13:11). According to a Tradition, the Messenger said, "Your Lord has gifts of His mercy for you

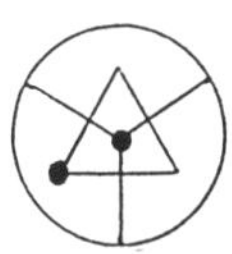

Temperance

throughout the days of your life so expose yourselves to them,"[1] that is, become prepared to receive by purifying the self of wrongdoing.

Temperance

The creative process in spiritual warriors' relationships with others is to perfect harmony *(bārī)* shaping a unique beauty (*muṣawwir*). They reach the point where they discover things in their relationship not known before. This discovery empowers them to produce and fashion that which has been discovered in perfect harmony, to work on the negative and bring form to the positive between and among themselves (*muṣawwir*). Then they will have created something positive that did not previously exist. Their friendship will grow in unity and strength.

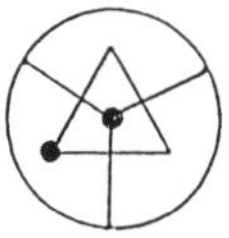

Temperance

Once they have become conscious of conceiving of the possibilities of the noble character traits, manifesting an aspect of courage, spiritual warriors then try in two ways to be a forgiver (*ghaffār*) of others. First of all, becoming repentant for their mistakes and secondly, concealing the faults of their friends from other people—hiding their inadequacies and mistakes—as they hope others will do with them. As a *ḥadith* says, "Those who cover over the imperfections of a believer, God will cover their imperfections on the Day of Judgment."[2]

Having completed stage one, awoken to their society around them by dying to their false self, spiritual warriors have entered the creative process to try to manifest His Signs upon the horizons in their relationships with others. That is, their goal is to create positive, healthy relationships with others of God's creatures.

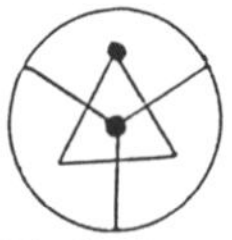

Wisdom

Repenting of their past mistakes, they now come to the second manifestation in the list of Most Beautiful Names that relates to will-power (*qahhār*). This will-power is also that of God's and not their own individual self. It is to subdue, kill, and humiliate their enemies within and without through a sense of wisdom. The greatest enemies within are their false self or ego and satanic temptations. Following this, they consciously try to control their irrational functions—inappropriate anger and desires—through the use of reason in their relationships with others.

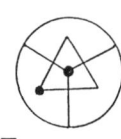

Anger arises from the instinctive desire to preserve the individual. Desires arises from the instinctive impulse to preserve the species. Their instinct manifests itself as avoidance of pain or attraction to pleasure. Both of these are life preserving qualities. They are appropriately expressed in their relationships with others. When they are regulated by the Law, reason can discipline and control them. If they are not regulated by the Law, they may fall victim to either one. Regaining control through reasoning will be more difficult. If they succeed in disciplining them through reason, their spirit will be revived.

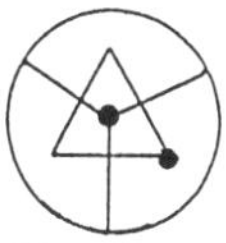

Courage

Once the animal instincts are under control of the reasoning function, they seek to give good to others (*wahhāb*) manifesting courage. When this giving comes from the sign of the Bestower (al-Wahhāb), nothing can prevent that good coming to us. If the Bestower gives good to another, nothing anyone can do can make it come back to them. When spiritual warriors manifest this, they do not expect to get anything in return. The servants of the Bestower are those through whom is given whatever God wishes, giving to those who are in need and who are worthy.

The master of the wise slave Luqman discovered Luqman's worth and became extremely attached to him so that he never received any delicacy without giving Luqman a share of it. One day, having received a watermelon, he gave Luqman the best part of it and Luqman devoured it with such apparent relish that his master was tempted to taste it. To his surprise he found it very bitter and asked Luqman why he had not told him this. Luqman replied that it was not for him, who lived on his Master's bounty, to complain if he now and then received disagreeable things at His hands.

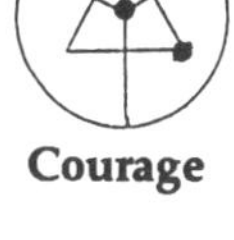

Courage

Manifesting their portion of the noble trait of being a provider (*razzāq*), expressing courage, spiritual warriors recognize that nourishment and sustenance come from God alone. Both the body and the self require nourishment. In a creative sense, nourishment of the self comes through gaining knowledge by which they then guide others. They use their power of speech in their relationships with others to direct people to the Straight Path by teaching them the Word of God. With their hands they give in charity. A Sign of the manifestation of being a provider is the dependence of others upon them.

At the beginning or while they are young, few moral-seekers have the spiritual insight to understand the depth of being a provider as this noble trait is little by little manifested through them. As they grow and have a family, only their immediate family is dependent on them for material or spiritual sustenance. Little by little as they continue to give in charity, to help others materially and spiritually, the number of people dependent upon them may grow perhaps into the thousands as it has for spiritual leaders throughout history.

As Rūmī points out, "Yea all the fish in the seas and all feathered fowl in the air above, all elephants, wolves, and lions of the forest, all dragons and snakes, and even little ants, yea, even air, water, earth, and fire draw their sustenance from Him, both winter and summer. Every moment this heaven cries to Him, saying, 'O Lord, quit not Your hold of me for a moment! The pillar of my being is Your aid and protection. The whole is folded up in that right hand of Yours.' And earth cries, 'Keep me fixed and steadfast, You who have placed me on the top of waters!' All of them are waiting and expecting to be provided for by Him. All have learned of Him to represent their needs. Every Prophet extols this prescription, 'Seek you help with patience and with prayer.' Seek aid of Him, not of other than Him. Seek water in the ocean, not in a dried-up channel.'"

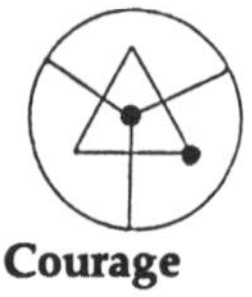

Courage

Next, in the creative unfolding of their relationships, spiritual warriors manifest the power to be an opener (*fattāḥ*) of all knots in their relationships to others, to remove sadness and depression from their hearts, and doubts from their minds through courage. The heart of the human being is God's house to which only God holds the keys. They stand at the door of al-Fattāḥ and knock in order to have the door to the heart opened to the treasury of mercy and generosity within. Manifestations of their intention to pray for the opening to the inner world appear when they help those who are weak in order to save themselves from those who are stronger; help those who have run into difficulties so that they will be helped when they fall; not hurt others because this is the key that locks the gate to mercy and blessings.

As they recreate their true self, they pray for knowledge and wisdom in dealing with others. This knowledge and wisdom they pray for is not formal knowledge but creative in the sense of how to approach God. The servants of the Knower (al-'Alīm) manifest wisdom towards others that is not learned from anyone, without studying or thinking.

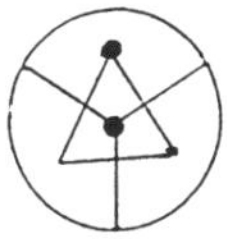

Wisdom

There is a well known story in this regard of Moses, peace be upon him, and the shepherd, showing the creativity of the shepherd as opposed to Moses who is reprimanded by God for having forgotten the importance of a creative approach when it is sincere. Once Moses came upon a shepherd who was praying, "Oh God, who chooses whom You will, where are You that I may become Your servant and sew your shoes and comb your hair, that I may wash Your clothes and kill Your lice and bring milk to You, O worshiped one, that I may kiss your little Hand and rub Your little Foot and at bedtime, sweep your little Room!!"

The shepherd was speaking in foolish words of love like this when Moses heard him. Moses asked, "Who are you addressing in this way?"

The shepherd said, "The One Who created us by whom this earth and sky were brought to sight."

Moses then began reprimanding the shepherd, saying, "What! Have you become so depraved. Indeed you speak like an infidel. What babble is this? What blasphemy and raving! Stuff some cotton in your mouth."

The shepherd felt ashamed and said, "Oh Moses, you

have closed my mouth and have burned my soul with repentance." He tore his clothes and heaved a heavy sign and turned towards the desert as he went on his way.

Suddenly a revelation came to Moses in which God said, "Moses, I sent you to unite people, not to separate them. You have turned My servant from me. To the point possible, do not set foot in separation. Of all things the most hateful to Me is divorce. I have given everyone a special way of acting. I have given to everyone a peculiar form of expression. I am not sanctified by praise. It is they who become sanctified. I do not look at the tongue and the speech. I look at the inward spirit and state of feelings. I gaze into the heart to see whether it be lowly though the words uttered be not lowly. I want burning, burning. Become friendly with that burning. Light up a fire of love in your soul. Burn thought and expression away."

From this story it becomes clear how God is the Knower of how spiritual warriors treat others and that serving God's purpose is to draw everyone to God—no matter what their position, status, ability or comprehension be. They learn not to be quick in judging others by their outer form alone but allow for the role of creativity, as well.

Chapter Three

Counseling to the Positive and Trying to Prevent the Development of the Negative

Next spiritual warriors will learn about the natural tension they have in counseling to the positive and avoiding the negative in their relationships with others. This tension is a part of their natural or instinctive nature or disposition (*fiṭrat Allāh*). It is an aspect of self that they share with animals. The two poles are attraction to pleasure and avoiding harm. Attraction to pleasure is a psychological expression of a biological need, namely, preserving the species. Avoidance of harm is also a psychological expression or state of a biological need or condition, namely, preserving the individual. Spiritual warriors know that preserving the species involves their relationships with others and therefore is ordered through laws relating to society, economics, and politics, among others. On the other hand, preserving the individual involves their relationship with self. The self is ordered through rules relating to psychoethics.

A third aspect of their basic instinctive nature as human beings is that of reason. It is this which separates us from animals. This function fully matures in us when they reach puberty. If their nurturing process has been healthy, they should be able to skillfully discipline and control the two instincts they share with animals—preserving the species (desire) and preserving the individual (anger).

At this stage, it is their reasoning ability which brings the first tension—that of attraction to pleasure versus avoidance of harm—to a higher level. The level is said to be higher for two reasons: first because it is a religious obligation clearly set forth in the Quran. This, then, implies the accountability of spiritual warriors to God for practicing it or failing to do so. Second, it can only be practiced with any kind of effectiveness when their reasoning abilities have been made operative. The sign of having attained a higher level of tension is the presence of the ability to fairly and justly 'command to the positive' (*amr bi'l ma'ruf*) and 'avoid the development of the negative' *(nahy an al-munkar*) or as referred to it in this work—counseling to the positive and avoiding the negative. Counseling to the positive is an extension of attraction to pleasure and preventing the development of the negative is an extension of avoiding harm.

Recognizing the tension between being a constrictor-expander (*qābiḍ-bāsiṭ*) as comparable to preventing the development of the negative and counseling to the positive, so also is being an exalter of truth (*rāfi'*) and abaser (*khāfiḍ*) of falsehood, an honorer (*mu'izz*) of their friends and humbler, dishonorer (*mudhill*) of their false self in their relations with others, looking at their relations as an arbiter (*ḥakam*) to foster objectivity and being just (*'adl*) and gentle (*laṭīf*) in their counseling to the positive and preventing the development of the negative. This results in becoming aware (*khabīr*) and conscious of their responsibilities in their relations with others to foster greater harmony and shape a unique beauty.

APPLICATION

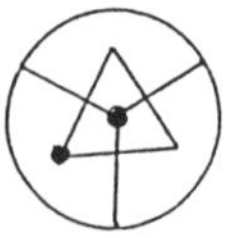

Temperance

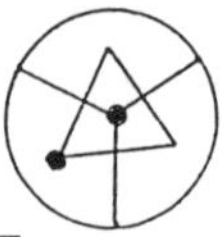

Temperance

At the beginning of the third stage, spiritual warriors face contradictions and paradoxes. These produce a tension within whereby they attempt to maintain a state of temperance as they move between fear and hope—fear of losing a friend, for instance, and hope for their relationship to continue. They move between being in a state of a constrictor (*qābiḍ*) and an expander *(bāsiṭ*).

Rūmī, tells of a prayer of a person between fear and hope, contraction and expansion. One night a man was crying, "God!" until his lips became sweet with the mention of His name.

Satan appeared and said, "Why now, chatterbox. Where is the answer, 'Here am I' to all this 'God' of yours? No answer is coming from the Throne. For how long will you grimly go on crying 'God'?" The man became broken-hearted and laid down his head to sleep. In a dream he saw Khidr in a green garden. "Look now," Khidr said, "why have you stopped from the mention of God? How is it you repent of having called upon Him?"

The man replied, "No answer of 'Here am I' is coming to me and I therefore fear that I have been repulsed from His door."

Khidr said, "God says that your cry of 'God' is itself My 'Here am I'. Your pleading and agony and fervor is God's Messenger. All your twistings and turnings to draw close to God are God's drawing you to Him that set free your feet. Your fear and hope are the lasso to catch God's grace. Under each 'God' of yours whispers many a 'Here am I'."

God occupied Moses, upon whom be peace, with the spiritual and the social. Though he was at God's command and altogether occupied with God, yet God occupied one side of him with social affairs for the general good. He occupied Khidr with Himself totally. He occupied Muhammad at first totally with Himself. Thereafter He commanded him, "Call the people, counsel them to the positive and help them try to prevent the development of the negative." Muhammad wept and lamented, saying, "Oh, my Lord, what wrongdoing have I committed? Why do You drive me from Your presence? I have no desire for people."

God said to him, "Muhammad, do not sorrow. I will not abandon you when you are helping people. Even in the midst of that occupation you shall be with Me. When you are helping people, not one moment of this hour you spend with Me, not one, will be taken from you. In whatever matter you are engaged, you will be in very union with Me."

Rūmī tells spiritual warriors, "Even when trouble befalls you, you should play close attention. You should look closely at the one who does us this ill turn. When you observe the ebb and flow of good and ill, you open a passage from misfortune to happiness. This is because you see that the one state moves you into the other—one opposite state generating its opposite in exchange. So long as you experience not fear after joy, how can you look for pleasures after pain? While you fear the doom of the angel on the left hand, you hope for the bliss of the angel on the right. May you gain two wings! A bird with only one wing is unable to fly."

If spiritual warriors listen to reason's advice and exhibit temperance and move between hope and fear, their 'self' is empowered to counsel to the positive and prevent the development of the negative. They learn to pray for patience during times of grief and suffering in their relations to others. They can turn a difficult experience into a positive one. Patience is to adopt a defensive wait and see position, falling back into God's Will as they let go of their own desires and expected results. It allows for a cooling off period from the situation of heightened tension. This prevents them from the harm of negative influences like becoming disoriented, confused, or depressed.

They counsel themselves to thank God for their blessings when they are in a state of expansion. They avoid becoming arrogant and proud towards their friends. Instead, they give freely to others of whatever they have, whether material or spiritual, and bring happiness to God's servants when they are in a state of expansion. They learn to maintain a balanced state, a state of centeredness in their relationships with others. This is to continue to do their duty and leave the rest up to God.

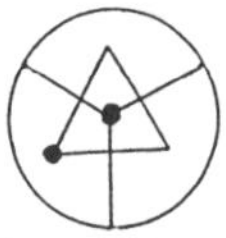
Temperance

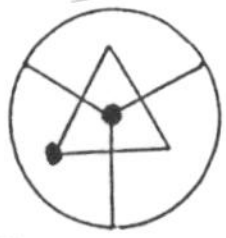
Temperance

When they counsel their 'self' in their relationships to manifest temperance by learning to exalt truth (*rāfi'*) and to prevent the development of falsehood (*khāfiḍ*), their relationships develop stronger roots. When their body bows down in prayer, their heart is as a garden and where there is a garden, there, bad friends are as weeds. When a liking for bad friends develops—those who counsel us to the negative and try to prevent the development of the positive—the very opposite of what good friends do for each other in accordance with God's command—they need to have the strength to exalt truth (*rāfi'*) and flee from them. Spiritual warriors have to uproot those weeds for if they attain full growth they will subvert them and their heart, as well. These 'weeds' turn them from the Straight Path, causing them to deviate from His Way.

Those who, within the potential of human imagination, raise their vision above things that are perceptible, who guide their will away from inappropriate anger and desire, are those whom God lifts up to the vision of the angels who are near to Him. Those who limit their vision to sensory things and manifest inappropriate anger and desire, which the animal kingdom shares with them but which animals express in an appropriate way, are the ones God abases. Whoever God abases, only God can exalt. In a sacred Tradition, God said to one of His friends, "As for your renouncing the world, you have earned your ease and comfort by it. As for your remembrance of Me, you have honored Me. But have you made a friend out of a friend of mine? Have you treated an enemy of mine as an enemy?"

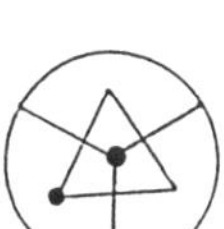

Temperance

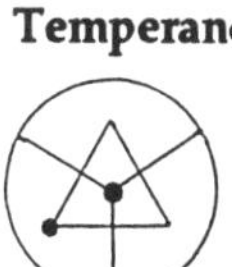

Temperance

When spiritual warriors counsel themselves to raise their friends to positions of honor (*mu'izz*) and humble themselves (*mudhill*), manifesting temperance, they counsel them to protect themselves against attributing falsehood to the Day of Judgment at the same time that they give counsel to those who are worthy of truth. They raise their friends to a position of honor in the same way that God has honored them, "*I honored the children of Adam*" and beckoned those so honored with, "*Oh soul at peace, return unto your Lord, well-pleasing! Enter your among My servants! Enter you My Paradise*" (89:27-30). The true sovereign (*malik*) is to be found in one who is free from the humiliation of physical needs, the dominance of inappropriate anger and desire, and the disgrace of ignorance. At the same time as spiritual warriors honor their friends, they humble ourselves before them as they strengthen their sense of temperance.

There is a story told in the Traditions of how an inappropriate sense of pride can interfere in the manifestation of this character trait. The Messenger, peace be upon him, was sitting in a gathering. His Companions formed a circle around him. In the midst of this, one of the Muslims who was very poor entered the room. Thus, according to Islamic custom, whenever a person enters a room, no matter what his position, he has to take the first free seat that he finds and not feel that because of his position, his place is such and such. As it would be, he sat next to a wealthy man. The wealthy man gathered up his clothes and sat to one side.

The Messenger noticed this. He turned to the wealthy man and said, "Were you afraid some of his poverty would rub off on you?"

"No, oh Messenger of God."

The Messenger then asked, "Were you afraid your clothes would be spoiled so you sat to one side?"

The wealthy man answered, "I must confess that I have erred. Now, in order to make up for this wrongdoing I have committed, I am willing to give half of all my wealth to this Muslim in order that he forgive me."

The poor man who had come into the room and been the reason for this conversation then said, "But I am not willing to accept."

Everyone in the group asked all at once, "Why not?"

The poor man said, "Because I am afraid that one day I will become very proud and behave towards a brother Muslim in the same way that he has behaved towards me."

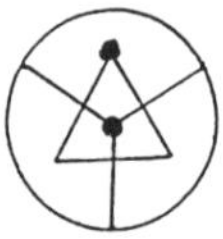

Wisdom

Continuing to counsel themselves to the positive and prevent the development of the negative, spiritual warriors intend to assume their portion of the noble trait of All-Hearing (al-Samī') through which they express wisdom. There is an amusing story related by Rūmī about someone who was hard of hearing but refused to admit it.

Just as people often perform works of devotion and set their hearts on being approved and rewarded yet those very works are in reality secret wrongdoing against God. What was thought to be pure is in fact not so at all.

An elderly person who was going deaf, but refused to admit it, was told that his neighbor had been taken ill. The deaf man said to himself, "With my hardness of hearing, how shall I understand what my sick and weak neighbor is saying. Yet, on the other hand, I have to go and see him. He is my neighbor. I know what I will do. I will guess what he is saying out of my own initiative. When I say, 'How are you, my poor suffering friend?' he will answer, 'I am fine,' or 'Quite well, thank you.' Then I will say, 'Thank God! What have you had to drink?' He will answer, 'A sherbet,' or 'Some bean soup.' Then I will say, 'Good health! Which doctor is attending you?' He will answer, 'So and so.' I will say, 'He brings good fortune. Since he has called on you, all will go well with you. I have tested his good fortune. Wherever he goes, every want is granted.'"

Having readied his answers in advance, the man went to call on his neighbor. "How are you?" he asked.

"Dying," the sick man said.

"Thank God!" cried the hard of hearing man.

Thereupon the invalid became anxious. He thought to himself, "What sort of thank God is this? He must have been my enemy."

The deaf man had made his guess but it had turned out wrong. He next asked, "What have you had to drink?"

The sick man said, "Poison."

"Good health!" cried the visitor, making the patient still more angry. "Which doctor is attending you?" the man asked.

The sick man answered, "The Angel of Death. Get out!"

"Cheer up," the man who was hard of hearing said, "He brings good fortune, thank God" and left. The sick man was in a much worse state when the man left than when he had come in.

Through manifesting their portion of the trait the All-Hearing, spiritual warriors learn to guard their tongue against backbiting others, and to listen closely to the recitation of the Word of God. With the positive trait of wisdom, they come to see what is not evident to the average mind combining penetration and keen practical judgment. They then try to orient others towards seeking their own perfection of self.

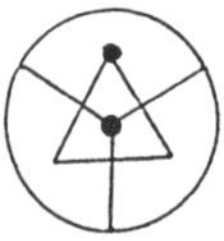
Wisdom

When they behold the Signs of God's creation to the extent that they come to know He sees them even if they do not see Him, they are expressing their portion of the sign the All-Seeing (al-Baṣīr). In reference to those who see and hear the Truth, God says in a Divine Tradition, "My servants come close to me with continuous devotion until I love them and when I love them, I become their ears with which they hear and the eyes with which they see and the tongue with which they speak and the hand with which they hold."

God calls Himself "the All-Seeing" to the end that His eye may every moment scare human beings from wrongdoing. God calls himself "the All-Hearing" to the end that they may close their lips against foul language. God calls himself "the All-Knowing" to the end that they may be afraid to plot wrong against those who have only done good to us.

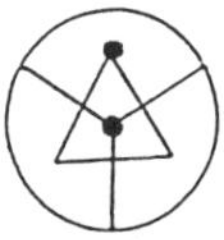
Wisdom

Working on their sense of wisdom, spiritual warriors try to bring truth and justice (*ḥakam*) to their relationships with others as the goal of their counseling to good and preventing the development of the negative. They practice this on themselves and in their relations towards others. When they are a true judge of themselves, they learn to judge others as they judge themselves and then traces of the Arbiter (al-Ḥakam) can then be seen within.

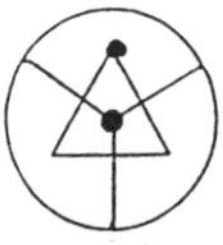
Wisdom

Learning to give rights in the right measure to those who have rights over them is to be just (*'adl*). In doing this, spiritual warriors counsel themselves and others to reason rather than irrationality by showing them how to place things in positions appropriate to them. Putting everything in its place is a manifestation of the Just (al-'Adl).

Once a gnat flew in from the garden and called on Solomon, peace be upon him, for justice, saying, "Oh Solomon, you extend your equity over *jinn* and the children of Adam. Fish and fowl dwell under the shelter of your justice. Where is the oppressed one whom your mercy has not sought? Grant me redress for I am much afflicted, being cut off from my garden and meadow haunts."

Solomon asked, "Oh seeker of redress, tell me from whom do you desire redress? Who, puffed up with arrogance, has oppressed you?"

The gnat replied, "The one from whom I seek redress is the wind. The wind has oppressed me. Through its oppression, I am in a grievous state. Through it I drink blood with parched lips!"

Solomon replied, "O sweet-voiced one, you must hear the command of God with all your heart. God has commanded me saying, 'Oh dispenser of justice, never hear one party without the other!' Until both parties come into the presence, the truth is never made plain to the judge."

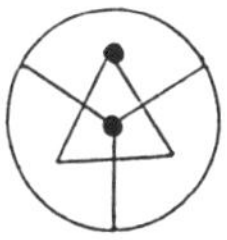

Wisdom

Spiritual warriors learn to be gentle *(laṭīf)* towards others, manifesting wisdom. They learn to counsel others to the positive, drawing them to accepting the truth through their own good qualities rather than through harshness, contempt, or fanaticism. These latter are to act in an extreme way and this is to go beyond the Straight Path. After practicing counseling their 'self' and others to the positive, the truth, and away from the negative, their reward given by God is to have their insight opened to inner beauty. They then relate to all of creation in a beautiful way so that each creature may express its inner beauty, as well.

In this way they come to realize that the creator of thought is more subtle *(laṭīf)* than a thought itself. For instance, an architect who designs and builds a house is more subtle than the house itself. He or she is able to design hundreds of such buildings, each different from the other. However, his or her ability can only be seen through the medium of a building, something that becomes part of the sensible world. Their qualities and attributes are like their thoughts, too subtle to appear except through some medium. They only appear when they act. No one can see their sense of mercy but when they forgive another who has wronged them, their mercy becomes visible. Their vengefulness, rightful or wrong, is too subtle to appear unless they act, for instance, by punishing a criminal who has broken the law. Then their attribute of being an avenger appears. The manifestation of their portion of the Subtle (al-Laṭīf) appears in how they relate to other people, their actions arising out of their inner qualities or attributes which are too subtle to be directly perceived.

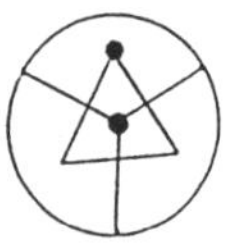

Wisdom

Attempting to attain consciousness, awareness manifesting the Sign the Aware (al-Khabīr), spiritual warriors counsel others to the same, gaining wisdom. They are told in the Traditions to become aware of what takes place in their body and their heart. Only testing themselves in this way will they become aware of the hidden things which could characterize their heart, namely, deception and treachery, preoccupation with things of this world, holding grudges while pretending to like someone, or pretending to be sincere. Consciousness of these negative traits within themselves and others comes through experiencing them in the irrational aspects of self. For spiritual warriors, it is to become familiar with their cunning ways and then control them with the rational faculty.

A jackal fell into a dye-pit and its skin was dyed of various colors. Proud of its splendid appearance, it returned to its companions and desired them to address it as a peacock. But they proceeded to test its pretensions, saying, "Do you scream like a peacock or strut about gardens as peacocks do?" It was forced to admit that he did not, whereupon they rejected his pretensions.

Another time a proud man who lacked food found an animal skin full of fat. He greased his beard and lips with it and called on his friends to observe how luxuriously he had dined. However, his belly was rumbling at this because it was hungry and he was undermining his chance of being invited to dinner by his friends. His belly cried to God and a cat came and carried off the skin of fat so the man's false pretenses were exposed.

Chapter Four

Developing the Moral Reasonableness of a Religiously Cultured Monotheist

Being a forebearer (*ḥalīm*) marks the beginning of spiritual warriors' moral reasonableness. The word *ḥilm*, from which it comes, is usually defined as patience or forbearance. But here, among the noble character traits, spiritual warriors extend the definition based on the role the concept played in history where it is described as moral reasonableness. And not just moral reasonableness, but that of a religiously cultured monotheist.

Being reasonable means not being extreme or excessive in their behavior towards others. They are moderate and fair, possessing sound judgment in the decisions they make. Being moral means they are conscious of the principles of right and wrong in their behavior. Being cultured means having integrated their knowledge, beliefs, and behavior in such a way that they are able to transmit their pattern to succeeding generations. They can summarize this concept of moral reasonableness by saying it is to seek justice for others but not for themselves. It is a person who holds back his or her natural instinct to a violent and emotional kind of anger; remains tranquil so that he or she not be easily moved by anger; does not lose control when a calamity strikes; is so in control of the self that requital of wrong-doing is slow in being manifested

The basis for *ḥilm* is the belief in the One God, the Creator of the universe. It is to counsel to kindness (*iḥsān*) in human relations with an emphasis on justice and the preventing of wrongful violence while counseling the self to abstinence and the control of passions. It includes concepts like forbearance, patience, and liberating the self from being moved and stirred up by the smallest provocation. This is the direction and orientation of the true morally reasonable person (*ḥalīm*). Such a person develops moral reasonableness because of his or her sense of guarding against the negative (*taqwā*). This is one of the main bases of spiritual chivalry (*javānmardī, murāwwah* or *futuwwah*).

Armed with moral reasonableness, spiritual warriors develop the power to generate what is right (*'aẓīm*) with others and conceal their faults (*ghafūr*) while they are thankful (*shakūr*) for recognizing their own faults. They extend their good qualities towards others (*kabīr*) without any thought of recognition by them as a preserver (*ḥafīẓ*) of their purified heart. They try to be a maintainer (*muqīt*) of balance and harmony in their relations because they are now morally obliged to be a reckoner (*ḥasīb*) of their own shortcomings.

Courage

APPLICATION

The potential for being a morally reasonable person (*ḥalīm*) can only be actualized through self-discipline. Once in Baluchistan a man went to a barber to tattoo his body with blue objects to ward off the evil eye. The barber asked, "What image do you want me to tattoo?" The man said, "Tattoo the figure of a raging lion. I was born under the sign of Leo so prick out a picture of a lion. Use lots of blue in doing it."

As soon as the barber began to stick the needle in the man, feeling a sharp pain in his shoulder-blade, he cried out in a seemingly brave tone, "Noble sir. I say, you are killing me. What sort of a figure are you tattooing?"

"Why, a lion just as you ordered," the barber answered.

"With which part did you begin?" the man asked.

"I began with the tail," the barber replied.

"Omit the tail," the man said. "The lion's tail and rump took my breath away. Let the lion be tailess and rumpless. The prick of the needle has made me feel faint."

The barber began to prick another part of the lion. The man cried out, "What part of the body is this now?"

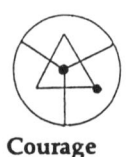

"This is the ear, my good man," said the barber.

"Let it be without ears."

The barber began another part and yet again the man yelled out, "What part is this now?"

"This is the belly of the lion, sir."

"Let him lack for a belly," the man said. "The picture is full enough already. What need for a belly?"

The barber was beside himself. He flung the needle to the ground crying out, "Whoever saw a lion without a tail, a head, or a belly? God Himself never created such a lion."

The man who had gone for the tattoo lacked courage which is essential as they bear the pain of self-discipline. They have to be forbearing in the pain that they suffer in order to discipline themselves. There is no growth without pain.

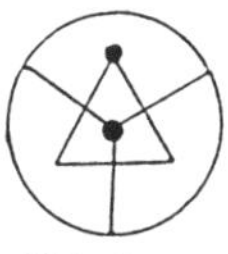

Wisdom

From their moral reasonableness comes the power to generate what is right in relating to others (*'aẓm*) through wisdom. This power arises from having cultivated an inner greatness, magnificence, and strength (*'aẓīm*). This inner greatness, magnificence, and strength comes from their dying to their false self. Only in the state of nonbeing can they effectively manifest moral reasonableness. Dying to their false self has been illustrated in the well-known story of the merchant and his parrot.

A merchant lived in Baghdad with his lovely, caged parrot. When he had to travel to India, he asked the parrot what gift he could bring for it. The parrot said, "When you see the wild parrots in India, tell them that I am yearning to join them but heaven has decreed that I remain a prisoner. Ask them to help me find the right guidance so that I not die separated from them. Say: 'Is it fair that I rot in bondage while you are free to fly wherever you want? Is this how friends help friends? Me in prison while you are in rose gardens? Remember me this friend of yours.'"

The merchant promised to give its message to the parrots in India. When he reached a remote area, he saw a number of parrots. He gave them the message whereupon one of the parrots began to tremble, fell down, and died. The merchant was dismayed to have caused such a tragedy.

When the merchant returned to Baghdad he was reluctant to tell his parrot what had happened, feeling he had been responsible for the death of the parrot. His parrot pleaded and he finally relented. He said when he gave the parrots the message, one parrot trembled, fell down to the ground and died.

His own parrot, upon hearing this, trembled, fell down in his cage and stopped breathing. The merchant was once again overwhelmed at what had happened. In his anger at himself for having told his parrot the story, he flung open the door to the cage, picked up his parrot and threw it out of the cage. The parrot gained life and flew to a branch of the tree. The merchant could not believe his eyes. He asked his parrot what counsel the Indian parrot had given it. His parrot said, "It bid me to give up my charming voice and my affection for my master since these were the things that had put me in bondage. By dying to itself, it said to me, 'Be dead as I am dead and be delivered, receive salvation.'" The parrot, then, had died to its false self and given up control to God whereby it was freed.

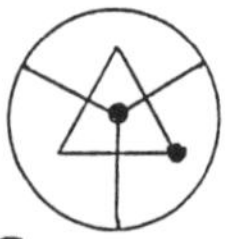

Courage

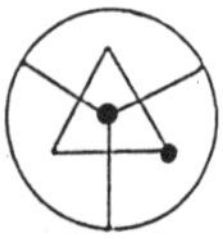

Courage

At the same time that they cultivate inner strength, spiritual warriors recognize their weaknesses and areas of vulnerability. Before they can acquire the following two traits, that of being forgiving, concealers of faults (*ghafūr*) and thankful (*shakūr*) towards others, they need faith. Faith precedes prayer. Taking prayer to be the prescribed prayer (*ṣalāt*), they compare them. The prescribed prayer is performed five times a day; faith is continuous. The prescribed prayer can be dropped for a valid excuse and may be postponed. Not so faith. Faith cannot be dropped for any excuse and may not be postponed. Faith without the prescribed prayer is beneficial. The prescribed prayer without faith confers no benefit. In their search for moral

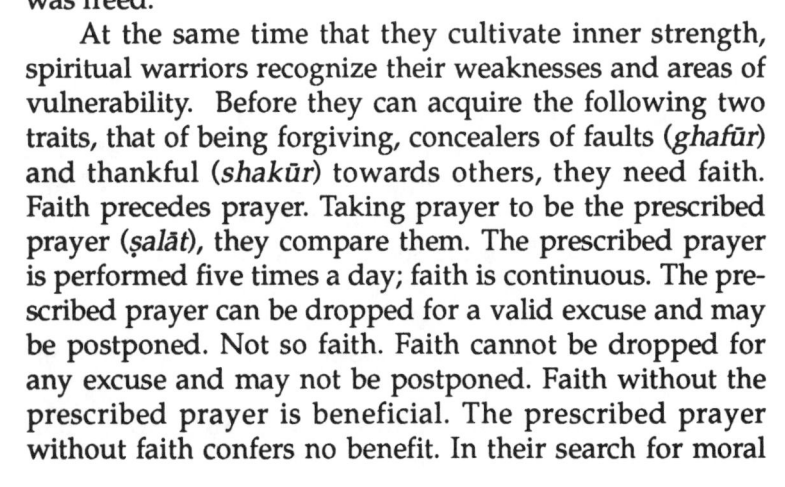

reasonableness, therefore, spiritual warriors must first find faith which is essentially none other than remembrance, consciousness, the opposite being forgetfulness or unconsciousness.

Forgetfulness is unbelief. Faith cannot exist without the existence of unbelief, for faith is the forsaking of unbelief. Therefore there must be unbelief which is then forsaken. Both of these are one and the same thing since one does not exist without the other. The prayer of hypocrites and the prayer of the various religions is of a different kind whereas faith does not change in any religion: its states, its locus, and so forth are invariable.

Expressing their new found sense of being morally reasonable (*ḥalīm*), spiritual warriors show compassion (*raḥīm*) towards believers, being a forgiver (*ghaffār*) of their wrongdoings towards others, thankful (*shakūr*) to the Magnificent (al-'Aẓīz), the Able (al-Qādir), the Loving (al-Wadūd), as they continue to ask for forgiveness again and again. Here, manifesting courage, they seek that their faults and those of all believers be concealed from the spiritual world.

In return for the sense of expansion and exuberance that follows, as morally reasonable, they express being thankful (*shakūr*), manifesting courage, one of the Most Beautiful Names which the human being contains in actuality and God metaphorically because God in His greatness and majesty is beyond a sense of thankfulness. This is why in reference to God, al-Shakūr is translated as "Rewarder of Thankfulness."

Expressing this Sign towards others, spiritual warriors repay any good done to them with a greater good. In thankfulness to God Who has provided them with everything that they need, they make use of what God has given them only for the purposes for which they were created—that is, to benefit creatures and not to harm them. Those who express this Sign see only good. They recognize that all good comes from God so they continuously express being thankful (*shakūr*).

Thankfulness is to hunt for and to shackle benefits. When spiritual warriors hear the voice of thankfulness, they get ready to give more. When God loves a servant, He afflicts him; if he endures with fortitude, He chooses him; if he is thankful, He elects him. Some people are grateful to God for His wrathfulness and some are grateful to Him for His graciousness. Each of the two classes is good; for thankfulness is a real antidote, changing wrath into grace. The intelligent and perfect human being is a person who is thankful for harsh treatment, both openly and in secret; for it is he whom God has elected. If God's will be the bottom of hell, by thankfulness His purpose is hastened.

On the other hand, a Sign of those who deny God's blessings, who are not thankful to Him with their hearts, is the fact that no matter what they have, it is not enough. Greed consumes them to have even more. Their blessings go unused and eventually rot and decay. They are people who they can see pass from one loss to another, from one disaster to another.

A sense of responsibility is also part of their moral reasonableness. They become detached and removed somewhat from their relationships, allowing for objectivity (*'alī*) while they are supportive and helpful to those around them as manifest in the story about the second Rightly-Guided Caliph, 'Umar.

During the time of caliph Umar there was a great fire in Madinah. Half the city caught fire from the flames. The people threw skins full of water and vinegar on the fire to no avail. The people ran to the caliph saying, "The fire will not be quenched by water."

The caliph said, "That fire is a Sign from God. It is a flame from the fire of your wrongdoings. Abandon water and distribute bread. Abandon greed if you are my people."

The people protested saying, "They have opened their doors to the poor. They have always been open-handed and charitable."

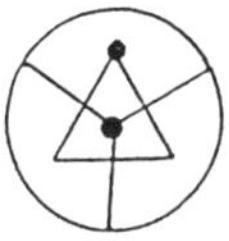
Wisdom

He said, "You have given bread out of habit but you have not opened your hands for God's sake. You have done so for your own glory—proudly and showing off—not because of a sense of piety and in humble submission." In other words, it is only giving as a religiously cultured person that one manifests a portion of the Highest (al-'Alī). Caliph 'Umar is expressing justice when he is apprehensive that a worse situation than a fire may fall on the people of Madinah so that he concentrates on trying to alleviate the situation.

Spiritual warriors sense God's greatness in relation to themselves as they manifest a sense of wisdom and reflect their portion of being 'great' (*kabīr*) when their attributes of perfection are not restricted to themselves but extend to others, as well. Any contact with another person can effect a transfer of some part of those qualities they have tried to perfect. Human perfection lies in reason, piety, and knowledge—formal and informal. Because of their piety, they become a model for others to follow. Their behavior becomes a pattern that others want to manifest. Others wish to learn logic and intuitive thinking from them. Prophet Jesus said of the expression of this Sign, "The one who knows and acts is the one who is called *kabīr* in the kingdom of heaven." This quality is a divine blessing whereby they grow inwardly and are perfected by God's hand alone. It is not without reason that the Quran says of God's Messenger, "*You have a good model in God's Messenger...*" (33:21).

Wisdom

With the development of their moral reasonableness they become aware of being a protector (*ḥafīẓ*) of others, keeping them from harm, however limited their portion of this trait may be.

Even the protection offered by Prophet Solomon was limited in scope. One day a nobleman ran into Prophet Solomon's judgment hall, his face pale with anguish, his two lips blue. Prophet Solomon asked, "What has happened to you?"

The man said, "Azrael, the angel of death has looked

upon me in great anger."

"Well, what do you want?" Prophet Solomon asked? The man said, "Command the wind to transport me to India. It may be that going there your slave will save his soul."

Prophet Solomon ordered the wind to bear him swiftly over the waters to the depths of India. The following day when his court was in session, Solomon spoke to Azrael saying, "Did you look on that true believer with such anger to drive him into being a wanderer far from home?"

Azrael said, "When did I look upon him with anger? I was astonished when I passed by and saw him for God had commanded me saying, 'This very day seize his spirit in India!' I said to myself in wonder, 'Even if he had a hundred wings, for him to be in India today is a far journey.'" The moral is to ask themselves from whom shall they flee? From themselves? Impossible. From whom shall they snatch themselves? From God? How impious. They seek refuge in God al-Ḥafiẓ, the Protector.

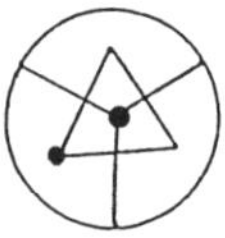

Temperance

Yet, when they express their portion of being a protector of other believers, their sense of protectiveness is so strong that not only are others around them protected against adversity, to a certain extent, but their minds and hearts are protected from negative thoughts and negative feelings, as well. They protect others by teaching them what God has provided that is good and what is harmful to them in the extension of the instinctive urge for survival.

Manifesting their individual portion of the Preserver, spiritual warriors avoid harms—both physical and spiritual—in their relations with others. Expressing temperance, they display no weakness when placed in a hostile situation to preserve the honor of others or in defense of the religious law. Expressions of this Sign include preserving and protecting the self from negative influences and rebellion against God's Commands. It is to help and protect others and to remember and preserve God's Word in

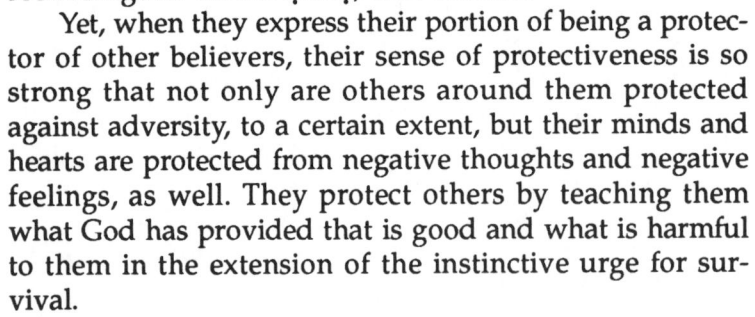

the Quran. If they meet a person whose inner and outer states, actions and words seem to be protected by some force, they are observing the manifestations of a portion of being a protector (*ḥafīẓ*). It is to have a sense of courage in its aspect of serenity within the self.

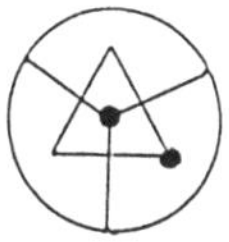

Courage

Spiritual warriors seek to understand what it means to be a 'maintainer' (*muqīt*) of others, as they manifest courage, reflecting the best model for their nurturing process. There was once a skinny person, feeble and contemptible, so contemptible to behold that even other contemptible forms looked on him with contempt and gave thanks to God, although before seeing him they used to complain of their own contemptible form. In addition, this person was angry in his speech and bragged enormously. He was in the court of the king and his behavior pained the minister who had raised him yet the minister swallowed it down. Then one day the minister lost his temper. "People of the court," cried the minister, "I picked this creature out of the gutter and maintained him. By eating my bread and sitting at my table and enjoying my charity and my wealth he became somebody. Now he has reached the point of saying such things to me!"

"People of the court," cried the man, springing up in the minister's face, "What he says is quite true. I was nourished by his wealth and charity until I grew up, contemptible and ignorant as you see me. If I had been maintained by someone else's bread and wealth, surely my form and stature and worth might have been better than this. He picked me out of the gutter; all I can say is 'Oh would that I were dust.' If someone else had picked me out of the gutter, I would not have been such a laughing stock."

The moral is that a person who is maintained at the hands of a parent who follows the way of God has a clean and chaste spirit. As morally responsible people they need to maintain those in their care through God's way and not their false way. He who is maintained at the hands of an impostor and a hypocrite and learns from him is just like the man in this story, contemptible and feeble, weak and with no way out, unable to make up his mind about anything, deficient in all his senses.

In furtherance of their moral reasonableness, spiritual warriors learn to take an accounting of things, showing their sense of courage. They learn to make good use of everything that God has provided while they assure the good management of God's blessings on His creation. They learn that their life is their temporary capital investment. Every day they spend out of their capital which at their death will be returned to its Owner where they will be rewarded for the capital gains they made and punished for their losses. When they are a reckoner (*ḥasīb*) of their deeds, they consider every moment of life as valuable. They spend it working for God's sake in caring for God's creation. They continuously remember God, thank God, and praise God, taking their actions each day into account so that they can begin a new day with their gains rather than losses.

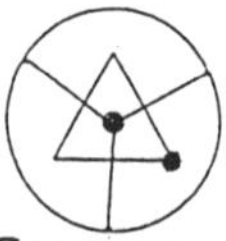

Courage

Just when they think they have attained some level, their accounting proves faulty. Once a scholar of Arabic grammar got on a boat. He asked the boatman with a self-satisfied air, "Have you ever studied grammar?'

"No," replied the boatman.

"Then half your life has gone to waste," the scholar said.

The boatman then felt very depressed but he said nothing for the moment. Presently the wind tossed the boat into a whirlpool. The boatman shouted to the scholar, "Do you know how to swim?"

"No," replied the scholar.

"In that case, scholar," the boatman remarked, "you have wasted all of your life because the boat is sinking in the whirlpool."

CHAPTER FIVE

USING THEIR SPIRITUAL POWER TO HELP OTHERS

Spiritual power (*jalīl*) and its manifestations in their relationships with others comes through the power to be generous (*karīm*), to be vigilant (*raqīb*), to comply with the requests of others (*mujīb*), to gain extensive knowledge of the world and self (*wāsi'*), and knowledge of God (*ḥakīm*), to develop a loving trust with others (*wadūd*), to perfect their moral reasonableness (*majīd*), to give life through knowledge (*bā'īth*), to witness the invisible and visible alike (*shāhid*), and to sense the truth (*ḥaqq*).

APPLICATION

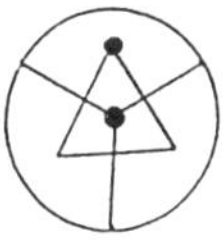

Wisdom

The Majestic (al-Jalīl) can be described as having might, dominion, knowledge, wealth, power, and the perfection of other attributes. It is to be wise, generous, compassionate, and spiritually powerful. When spiritual warriors manifest their portion of the Majestic (al-Jalīl) they are empowered to teach others that everything depends on God's Will. This is to include life, death, being, becoming, gain, and loss. Manifesting a portion of the Majestic (al-Jalīl), they manifest a sense of wisdom to whom they relate helping them reconcile differences of opinion through mutual assistance.

Once an ant saw a pen writing on a piece of paper. It whispered this mystery to another ant saying, "The pen drew wonderful pictures of roses and lilies and carnations."

The second ant said, "It is the finger that is the artist. The pen is just an instrument."

A third ant joined them and said, "No. It is the work of the arm. The power of the slender finger that drew those flowers comes from the arm."

Finally the leader of the ants joined in the conversation and said, "Don't think that this power comes from the physical form which becomes unconscious in sleep and decays at the time of death. Only reason and the spirit can cause the fingers to move. And that spiritual power comes from God the Majestic (al-Jalīl)."

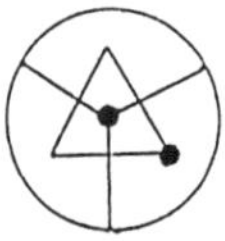

Courage

There is a Tradition (*ḥadith*) which describes the next Sign, the Generous (al-Karīm), an aspect of courage. The Messenger said, "The grapevine is characterized as being generous because, unlike the date palm, its fruit is delicious, picking it is simple, reaching it is easy, and it has no thorns or other causes of harm." To manifest their part of the Generous is to act in accordance with God's generosity. The Quran says, "*Oh people! What beguiles you from your Lord, the Generous, Who created you then made you complete, then made you in the best of states?*" (82:6-7).

Once there was a bedouin who had a dog that he dearly loved. The dog was dying and its master was beside himself. A passer-by asked, "For whom are you wailing and crying?"

"I am crying for my dog. It was a good tempered beast," said the bedouin. "See, he is dying there by the road. He was my huntsman by day and my watchman by night, sharp of eye, a fine trapper, alert in driving off thieves."

"What's wrong with him then?" the man asked. "Has he been wounded?"

"No," said the bedouin. "Hunger has brought him to this state."

"Then be patient," the passer by urged. "Bear up with this pain and agony. God's grace rewards the patient." Then he saw that the bedouin was carrying a full sack. He asked, "What's in the sack?"

The bedouin said, "Just bread and a few other scraps left over from last night's dinner. I'm taking them along with me to strengthen my body."

"Then why don't you give some bread and scraps to the dog?"

"Ah," the bedouin said, "my love and generosity do not

extend that far. When you are traveling you have to pay a lot for bread whereas the water from the tears that I am shedding is free."

This bedouin, clearly, is not manifesting the sign of a generous (*karīm*) person as exemplified in the Generous (al-Karīm)

It is said that an atheist wanted Abraham to invite him to dinner. Abraham said, "If you submit yourself to God, I will ask you to be my guest." The atheist went away. God then said in a revelation to Abraham, "Oh Abraham! You will not give this man dinner until he leaves his own religion! They have been giving him his provisions for seventy years in spite of his disbelief. If you had given him dinner tonight and not attacked him, how would you have lost anything?"

After this revelation, Abraham sought out the atheist and invited him to dinner. The man then asked why he had don so. When Abraham related what had happened, the atheist said, "If your God is so generous to me, then accept me into your religion!"[1]

As servants of the Generous, they are not satisfied with themselves until they are able to give or to help others. They do not seek thanks or recognition for what they do. As a result, further demands are made upon them. This is proof that God has accepted the services they have performed for others. The dangers of those who manifest this sign is to tire or to become proud of what they are doing. The dangers of those who do not manifest this Sign, who are in need, are hopelessness and doubt. They should neither doubt God's mercy nor his generosity. When they who are conscious of God the Generous and they endeavor to manifest the portion of this sign that is theirs, they help those in need to understand God's mercy and generosity.

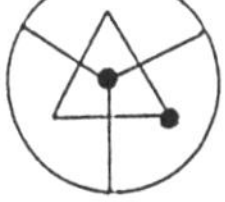
Courage

Being vigilant (*raqīb*) is to manifest courage in facing two enemies within the self: satan and one's ego in their relationships with others. It is vital to recognize these enemies who lead to negligence and disobedience. Those who are able to manifest a portion of this Sign are conscious and self-controlled.

Once there was a lion, a wolf, and a fox who joined together for a hunt. They managed to catch a mountain ox, a goat and a fat rabbit. Although the lion was ashamed to be seen with the wolf and the fox, he counseled himself to join with them out of pure generosity for he would have succeeded very well on the hunt without them. Meanwhile, the wolf and the fox were waiting for the majestic lion to divide up the spoils of the hunt in a fair and just manner. The lion, however, asked the wolf to perform this task, to divide up the catch.

The wolf, whose hunger pangs had reached the limit, said, "King of the beasts, the wild ox is your share. I shall have the goat and the fox should take the fat rabbit."

The lion was enraged by the division. He said to the wolf, "How dare you speak like that. With me present you speak of me and you!" The lion with one stroke killed the wolf because it had not passed away in the presence of the king of the beasts.

The lion then turned to the fox and said, "Divide up the catch and let us eat breakfast."

The clever fox said, "Best of kings, the ox is for your breakfast, the goat for your lunch and the fat rabbit for your dinner."

The lion was pleased with this and said, "Fox, you have lit the torch of wisdom. What an admirable division you have made. Where did you learn this?"

The fox answered, "From what happened to the wolf." The fox then said to himself, "Thank goodness the lion called me after the wolf. If he had called on me first, I would be where the wolf is now."

Whereas the lion lacked the quality of vigilance, the fox was clearly receptive to it. The fox also expresses gratitude that it was put in the world when it was. For spiritual warriors it is to be grateful that they were created after the peoples of old so that they hear of the punishments He has given to past generations, so that once they know what befell the wolf, they, like the fox, can be more vigilant.

There is a Tradition, "When half the night has passed, God will descend to earth and cry, 'You that ask, you shall be answered; you that crave pardon, shall be pardoned; and you that petition, your petitions shall be granted. But all who sleep the sleep of negligence will miss the promised blessing.'"

Spiritual warriors become very sensitive to the needs of others and are empowered to respond to them. The Messenger did not conquer Makkah and the surrounding lands because he was in need of them. He conquered them in order that he might give life to all people. His is a hand which is accustomed to giving. It is not accustomed to taking. When they learn to manifest their portion of the Majestic (al-Jalīl) and the Generous (al-Karīm), spiritual warriors develop the power to meet the requests of others (*mujīb*). Manifesting a part of responding to the prayer of others (*mujīb*) as their sense of courage, is reflected in their response to the Quranic verse, "*Therefore, the beggar drive not away*" (93:10), in other words, respond to his or her prayers.

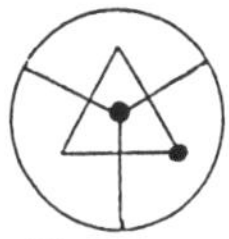

Courage

In dealing with others, spiritual warriors develop the power to gain knowledge of the world and their 'self' in terms of disposition (*wāsi'*). Through it they manifest an extensive, all-inclusive wisdom and a disposition that no longer includes fear of poverty, reaction to the envious, nor greed.

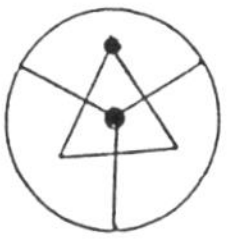

Wisdom

To be wise (*ḥakīm*) is also to manifest wisdom reflecting the most sublime and highest form of knowledge which is other than formal knowledge in their relationships with others. Only those who know God are considered to have this quality irregardless of their level of intelligence or eloquence in speech. The Quran says, "*Whoever is given wisdom is given a good deed...*" (2:269).

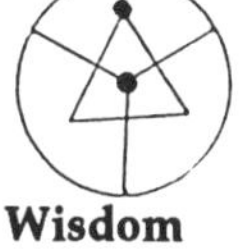

Wisdom

There are many Traditions recorded in regard to this Sign:

"The beginning of wisdom is the fear of God."

"The astute person is the one who judges the self and works for that which is after death while the incompetent subordinates himself to his passions and hopes in God."

"That which is little but sufficient is better than that which is plentiful but distracts."

"The one who awakes in the morning healthy in his body, secure in his household, and has his daily bread is as if the world belongs to him."

"Be pious and you will be the most devout of all people; be content and you will be the most thankful of all people."

"Speech is the cause of misfortune."

"A part of the beauty of one's Islam is the avoidance of that which does not concern him."

"The happy one is the one who is instructed by the example of another. Silence is wisdom, but there are few who accomplish it."

"Contentment is a wealth that will not be consumed."

"Perseverance is half of faith; certainty is the whole of faith."

As they increase their spiritual power, spiritual warriors learn to desire for others what they desire for themselves. They learn not to remain angry, full of hatred or resentment for harm done to them. The Messenger said after the Battle of Uhud when his teeth had been broken and his face bloodied, "Oh God, guide my people for they do not know." In a Tradition, the Messenger had said to 'Alī, "If you want to be closer to God than those already close to Him, then make up with those who have broken relations with you, give to those who excluded you, forgive the ones who wronged you."[2]

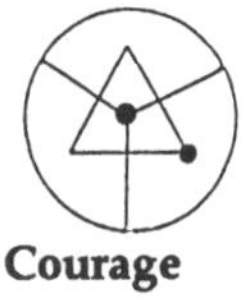

Courage

The goal of the heart of those who manifest the Sign of loving (*wadūd*), furthering their sense of courage, is to seek God's love alone. Based on a Tradition, "When God loves a servant of His, He says to Gabriel, 'I love this servant of Mine. Love him/her also.' Then Gabriel says to the heavens, 'Oh all those who are in the heavens, God loves this servant, so love him/her, too.' All that exists in the heavens comes to love him/her. The love of that servant is proposed to the creatures of earth and they also love him/her.

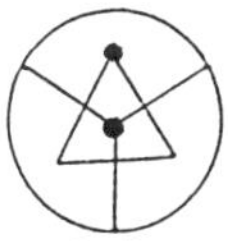

Wisdom

Spiritual power also brings glory which consists of noble essence, goodness of actions, and generosity in giving as they develop courage and their sense of honor. The Glorious (al-Mājid) is to combine the qualities of the Majestic (al-Jalīl), the Bestower (al-Wahhāb) and the Generous (al-Karīm).

Little by little spiritual warriors develop the power to take people out of ignorance of Reality, which is the worst kind of death, and help them be reborn in knowledge of God, the noblest form of life. When a person lays a trap and by cunning catches little birds in his trap so as to eat them and sell them, that is called cunning. But if they lay a trap so as to capture an untutored and worthless hawk, which has no knowledge of its own true nature, and to train it to their forearm so that it may become noble and taught and tutored, this is not called cunning. Although it may outwardly appear to be cunning yet it is known to be the very height of bounty and generosity, restoring the dead to life, converting the base stone into a ruby, making the dead sperm into a human being and far more than that. If the hawk knew for what reason people seek to capture it, it would not require any bait. It would search for the trap with soul and heart and willingly fly on the hunter's arm.

Overcoming and helping others to overcome ignorance of Reality is to give life to the dead. They are revived with a blessed life. Whoever acquires knowledge and does not practice it resembles someone who ploughs his land and leaves it unsown. Once they understand that they die as they lived and will be resurrected as they died, that they will reap whatever they have sown here in the Hereafter, they then direct their efforts towards sowing good deeds much as they would sow seeds in the earth. This work is to manifest an aspect of the Resurrector (al-Bā'ith), manifesting temperance.

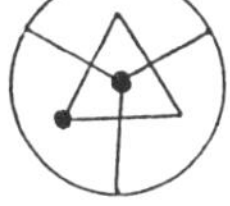

Temperance

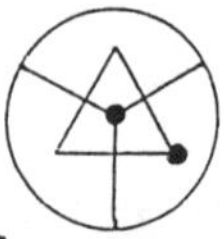

Courage

To this point spiritual warriors have learned about two types of knowing: the intuitive knower of the visible, external world (*'alīm*) and of the invisible, internal aspects of the world (*khabīr*). The third is that of the witness (al-Shāhid), expressing courage. Manifesting their portion of this quality, spiritual warriors take control of their life with courage in order to develop reason in coming to know both the external and internal worlds as they bear witness to the truth of everything having come from God.

A young man said to his father, "The pompous and heart rending sermons of the religious scholars make no impression upon me because I do not find their practice in conformity with their teachings. They teach me to abandon the world but they themselves run after it. Why should one teach mankind and forget one's own self? A religious scholar who runs after money has lost his own way. How can he show the right path to others? Can the drowsy teach others to keep awake?"

His father replied, "It is not wise to turn your attention away from the advice of men of learning merely on account of some of their weaknesses, accusing them of contradiction in their words and deeds and remaining excluded from the benefits of knowledge. If you shut your eyes, the sun cannot show you the way."

Maḥmūd Shabistarī, a 13th century mystic, acts as a witness (*shāhid*) when he says in his *Gulshan-i-rāz*:

> Know that the world is a mirror from head to foot
> In every atom are a hundred blazing suns
> If you cleave the heart of one drop of water
> A hundred pure oceans emerge from it
> If you examine closely each grain of sand
> A thousand Adams may be seen in it
> In its members a gnat is like an elephant
> In its qualities a drop of rain is like the Nile
> The heart of a barley-corn equals a hundred harvests
> A world dwells in the heart of a wheat seed
> In the wing of a gnat is the ocean of life

In the pupil of the eye, a heaven
What though the grain of the heart be small
It is a station for the Lord of both words to dwell
therein.

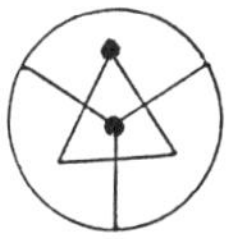

Wisdom

Finally their development of spiritual power culminates in expressing a sense of wisdom as spiritual warriors manifest their portion of the Truth (*ḥaqq*) whereby they see their 'self' as false and God alone as the Real. They annihilate self so that only God's Will remains operative. For the believers, faith and words are true aspects of the Real, if they relate to the permanent causal existence because these are what are constant and alive. The servants of the Truth (al-Ḥaqq) are not false in either their actions or words. They are aware of the Truth at all times in all circumstances. The Truth is always present and constant for them through their manifestation of unity and oneness.

There is a well-known parable about Solomon and Queen Bilqis (the Queen of Sheba or Saba). Their relationship is symbolized by a paralyzed child.

"Tell me, Solomon," Bilqis said, "we are both strong and healthy—why is our child (relationship) not healthy as well? Is there no remedy for his affliction? Let us try to find one. The next time Angel Gabriel brings you a message, ask him to read and tell you all that is written about this secret in the divine tables of fate. Perhaps there is a chance for our child to be cured—who knows?"

Solomon agreed and when the angel appeared, he told him of his wish. Gabriel went away but soon returned with greetings for Solomon from the Creator. He said, "Know that two things are necessary if your child is to regain its health and both are most precious and rare in this world: the husband must tell the truth to his wife and the wife to her husband..."

When Bilqis heard this, she was very happy and said, "Question me, Solomon, so that I can answer as God Wills."

Solomon thought for a while; then he asked, "Your

beauty is the target of all eyes. But you yourself, did you ever feel passion for anyone except me?"

"May the evil eye remain far from you!" replied Bilqis. "For me you are more radiant than the sun and superior to everybody in everything—not only through your youthful beauty, your kindness and your tenderness! You offer your guests a paradise on earth and you yourself are the guardian of this paradise. Whatever exists down here, visible or hidden, belongs to you, for the seal of your power as a Prophet is to preserve this world...and yet! In spite of your youthful beauty, in spite of your kingdom and your state of grace, it has happened to me that, looking at one or the other youth, I did not remain free from desire..."

No sooner had Bilqis allowed this confession to escape her lips than the child beside her—what a miracle!—lifted his helpless little hands, stretched them out towards her and called, "Look, Mama, look! They move!"

Profoundly happy, Bilqis turned to Solomon and said, "My Lord, good and wise, master over demons and fairies: now, for the sake of their child, you must answer my question, if it does not disturb you—so that his legs may be cured through your reply to me, just as his arms were cured through my answer to you. You possess more treasures on this earth than anyone else; tell me whether, in spite of your riches, you have ever coveted your neighbors possessions?"

Whereupon Solomon replied, "You are right. No man ever possessed so much power, so many treasures between heaven and earth as I. Yet I have to confess that I am desirous of ever more and often look secretly at the hands of those who come to pay their respects to me, wondering how many presents they are bringing..."

The words had hardly been spoken when the river of life rushed into the legs of the little one, who happily began to kick and to crawl. Through God's grace, he had been cured because his parents had not hidden from each other the truth about themselves.

The child of Solomon and Bilqis can be seen as other

than a physical person. No relationship, least of all their relationship with God, can survive in the darkness of lies and deceit. The relationship, like the young child in the story, will be paralyzed, without movement, without growth, without love. Without truth between two people there can be no trust. Without trust there can be no real relationship.

Chapter Six
God's Trustee

Trust comes from the verse, "*We offered the trust to the heavens and the earth and the mountains, but they refused to carry it and were afraid of it and the human being carried it...*" This trust is a task that the morally conscious never forget. The reasoning is that human beings have come into the world for a particular task. And that is their purpose. If they do not perform it, it is as if they have done nothing.

Consider for a moment how many tasks the heavens and the earth perform. The heavens convert common stones into rubies and diamonds. They make mountains into mines of gold and silver. They cause the seeds in the earth to germinate and spring into life. The earth receives the seeds and bears fruit. It accepts and reveals hundreds of thousands of marvels such as can never be fully told. They do all these things yet they do not do the one task that human beings are responsible for and that is to carry out the trust. By doing this, human beings become morally responsible people.

Someone may say, "'Well, I may not perform that task but I do so many others.' The answer is you were not created for the other tasks. It is as if you were to buy a sword of priceless damascene steel and use it as a butcher's knife to cut up meat saying, 'I will not let this sword be idle. I am putting it to use.' Or it is as if you were to take a bowl made of gold and cook turnips in it while for a single gram of gold you could buy hundreds of pots."

Therefore, it is important for spiritual warriors to serve the task for which they have been sent and not to be satisfied with themselves until they do so. Their task here is to understand that task of trusteeship which has instilled within them a morality, which they call being the moral reasonableness of a religiously cultured monotheist (*ḥalīm*).

The sixth stage revolves around the idea of trusteeship which is the basic foundation for solid relationships. When they have awoken to the desire to grow close to God, embarked upon the creative process of transforming their relationships, counseled themselves to the positive and tried to prevent the development of the negative, and been given spiritual power, spiritual warriors enhance their reasoning and thinking abilities through understanding their portion of being God's trustee (*wakīl*). From that they strengthen their thoughts (*qawī/matīn*) to defeat the enemy within and without so that their relationships can flourish. Through this strength, they are able to become friends with the friends of God *(walī)* and overcome their enemies, being praiseworthy *(ḥamīd)* in their deeds and leaving aside the negative*(ḥamīd)*, accounting of their wrongdoings (*muḥṣī*) and repenting for them, seeking understanding of their origins (*mubdi'*) and their end (*mu'id*).

APPLICATION

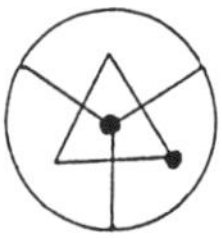
Courage

The basis for their relationship with God is that of trust, "*We offered the trust to the mountains and only the human being accepted.*" As human beings, they then become the trustee *(wakīl)* of God for nature and the universe, manifesting courage. Ibrahim Adham once made known in Baghdad that he was planning to journey to Makkah. One man on hearing the news rushed to see him, begging to be taken and offering to carry all the provisions for them both. When Ibrahim heard this, he replied, "I shall be your companion on the way but only on the condition that they carry no provisions and that if anyone offers us something, they refuse it reciting the verse, '*And whosoever trusts in God, God will suffice him*'" (65:3).

As trustees spiritual warriors try to avoid excessive ambition, miserliness, competitiveness, fear, and imagination while they manifest mercy, compassion, and love. They act as God's vicegerents as they safeguard nature and His creatures.

They manifest this quality of trusteeship, then, at various levels or stages. First with their words they say to another, "You can trust me with your secret." If their words are not confirmed by their reason, they soon forget that they have even made such a promise. Their knowledge, faith, experience, and conviction are weak. Their claim is verbal only. Soon another cause intervenes and sways us to telling that person's secret to another. What is forgotten is the basic cause of manifesting a portion of God the Trustee (al-Wakīl) because they see themselves as independent of God. They may even continuously recite ya-Wakīl but they do so in hopes of God's mercy saving them on the Day of Judgment and not because they are prepared to practice what they are saying. At this stage they cannot be said to be trustworthy in their relations with God much less in their relations with other people.

Whatever is seen in them is the reflection of God much like how the reflection of the moon appears in water. Often, forgetting this, spiritual warriors turn to another for help. At this stage, they become conscious of the fact that to God alone should they trust.

A benefactor may give spiritual warriors a cap but God gives their mind the power of the senses or a benefactor may give them clothes whereas God created their form. They may receive gold from another but their hand which receives and their mind which counts is from God. They may be given a horse but God provides their reason to guide the horse, or a lamp but He gives them their eyes, or sweets but He gives them their appetite, or a pension but He gives them their very life and being. Whatever rightful thing another provides them with from themselves ultimately comes from God including the generosity of the person so giving. With their trust in God alone they become like a guide to the highest qualities the human being can attain and this is the very sign of their humanness.

At the second stage, spiritual warriors are convinced by reason or revelation that they are God's vicegerents on earth and when they are entrusted with a duty which they faithfully carry it out in their words or actions. They are fully conscious that God has knowledge of the needs of His creatures; the power and ability to satisfy those needs; freedom from stinginess and love and mercy for all creatures. As God does not deprive spiritual warriors of what is good for them even though they themselves may be incapable of distinguishing between what is beneficial and harmful. At this stage they are rational trustees but not trustees through faith. Here reason dominates their heart.

At the third and highest level, their responsibility for the trusteeship has penetrated their hearts and become a part of their faith. The Sign is contentment. At this stage their body is in servitude to God and their heart is in the state of contentment. This is what the Messenger manifested even before this messengership when he was known among the people of Makkah as the Trustworthy (al-Amīn).

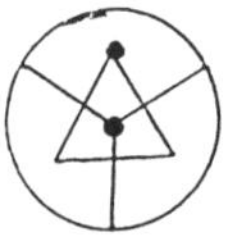

Wisdom

As trustees in faith—verbally, mentally, and emotionally—they become strong (*qawī*) enough to be able to overcome worldly ambition, inappropriate anger or desires, negativity, and satanic temptations as they relate to others on a higher plane. An intense form of strength (*mat¡n*) accompanies this which gives firmness to the strength. This firmness is then operative in defending the truth and holding fast to their belief.

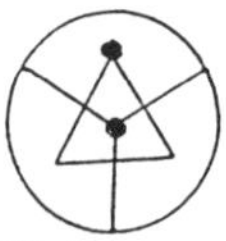

Wisdom

Manifesting a part of al-Qawī al-Matīn, aspects of wisdom, spiritual warriors are strengthened by words that lead them towards the Straight Path but their receptivity depends upon the amount of Grace He has given them. Strength and firmness, then, are preceded by Grace. When they err and become conscious of the fact that they are erring—"*For the human being was created a weakling*" (4:32)—they are receiving, the Grace of God—a pure gift, like a leaping spark of fire. When well received—that is, when they respond to it through consciousness and awareness—they nurse the spark, increasing its energy. The spark is their faith which increases when they nurture it with consciousness. From being a weakling, they move to "*Surely you are a mighty morality*" (68:4).

If God commands an army to attack a certain area and destroy it, so they will do; if He commands a single soldier to seize an area, he, too, will succeed. God sent a gnat against Nimrod and destroyed him. He sent a flock of birds against Abraha and Abraha was defeated. Equal in the eyes of those who manifest the signs of strength and firmness are a penny, a dollar, a lion and a cat. If God blesses a penny, it will do the work of a thousand dollars. If God withholds His blessings from a thousand dollars, it will not do the work of a penny. So, also, if God commissions a cat to destroy a lion as the gnat or mosquito destroyed Nimrod or if He commissions the lion, all lions will tremble before it. In the same way the furnace becomes "*coolness and safety,*" a bed of roses for Abraham because God's Grace had not determined that the fire consume him. In other words, when spiritual warriors realize all things are from God, all things become one and the same thing. It is then that their strength can match the strength of any enemy.

Understanding this principle of strength requires a receptiveness within. This is the root of the matter. If a thousand thieves come from without, they cannot open the door to their 'self' without a fellow-thief within. Listen to a thousand words from without, yet if there is none to confirm them within, they profit not. So, too, with a tree. If there is no freshness in its roots even though you were to pour a thousand buckets of water on it, it will absorb nothing. There must be freshness in the roots—receptiveness within the self—for the water to nurture it.

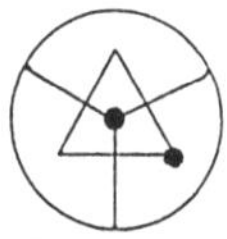
Courage

The next step for spiritual warriors who are God's trustees is to try to become a Friend (al-Walī) of God. When out of loneliness they fall into despair, they become radiant as the sun under the shadow of a true friend. When they seek the friend of God, God Himself becomes their Friend. They avoid strangers but not a friend. A fur coat is for winter, not for the summer. As they join their thoughts with a true friend, their thoughts will increase in their light and the road will become more clear as they manifest wisdom in its aspect of fidelity.

It is their false self or ego which, in control, can bring human beings down to a stage lower than that of animals. It is their ego or false self which veils them from their true self. The more precious and noble that true self be, the greater does their ego veil it. The veils can only be removed with great struggle.

The struggles and strivings of spiritual warriors are of various kinds. The greatest striving is to choose to mingle with friends who have turned their faces to God and turned their backs on this world. There is no more difficult striving then this—to sit with righteous friends. The very sight of them dissolves and negates the ego. It is for this reason that they say that when a snake has not seen a human being for forty years, it becomes a dragon. That is, because it sees no one who would be the means of dissolving its false self, its false self grows from being just a snake to becoming a dragon.

God said, "Peace be upon you, Prophet!" That is to say, "Peace is upon you and upon every human being." If this had not been the intention of God, the Prophet would not have countered Him and said, "Upon us and upon all God's righteous servants." For if peace had been intended solely for him, he would not have assigned it to righteous servants.

If spiritual warriors speak well of another, the good words reverts again to them and in reality it is they themselves that they are praising and applauding. It is like a person who sows his garden with flowers and aromatic herbs. Whenever he looks out, he sees flowers and aromatic herbs and is always in Paradise inasmuch as he has formed the habit of speaking well of other people. Whenever spiritual warriors engage themselves in speaking well of another, that person becomes their friend. When they remember them, they bring to mind a friend and bringing to mind a friend is like flowers and a flower-garden. It is refreshment and repose. But when they speak ill of another, they become hateful in their eyes. Whenever they remember them and their image comes before them, it is as though a snake or a scorpion, a thorn or a thistle had appeared in their sight.

Since they are able night and day to see flowers and a flower-garden, why should they go about amidst thorns and snakes? They should learn to love every person so that they may always dwell amongst flowers and a flower-garden. When they are an enemy of every person, the image of their foes appears before them and it is as if day and night they are going about amidst thorns and snakes.

Whatever they do to other people, whenever they make mention of them whether for good or ill, all that reverts to themselves. "*Whose does righteousness, it is to his own gain and whoso does evil, it is to his own loss*" (41:46). And "*whoso has done an atom's weight of good shall see it and whoso has done an atom's weight of evil shall see it*" (99:7-8).

When friends have seen very well into one another here below, when they come to be raised up in the other world, having become very familiar, they will quickly recognize one another. Knowing how they were together in the world of mortality, their reuniting will be with joy because they may all too quickly lose a friend. It may have happened that in this mortal world they have become a friend of some person and then on account of a single shameful action, that person vanishes from their sight and they lose him completely. Suddenly that person's form changed into a wolf for them. The very same person they saw formerly as a friend, they now see as a wolf for all that his actual form has not been changed. By that one accidental motion they lost their friend. Tomorrow when they are gathered together and their present form is changed into another, since they never knew that person well and never penetrated thoroughly into his essence, how are they going to recognize him? They must overpass the good and bad qualities which are present temporarily in every person and enter into the other's very essence, seeing exceedingly clearly that these qualities which people bestow upon one another are not their original qualities. This is truly seeing and knowing.

At the same time, they should test their friend so that in the end they may not have cause to regret. God said, "Begin with yourself. If the self makes claim to servanthood, do not accept its claim without making trial of it." Before drinking their water, people first smell the water and then they taste it. They are not satisfied simply to look at it. For it may be that the appearance of the water is perfectly good but the taste and smell of it are infected. This is an examination to test the purity of the water. Then, after the test has been completed, people apply the water to their faces.

Once a person becomes a Friend of God, the picture is very different than they would normally assume. It is related that Jesus, peace be upon him, was wandering in the desert when a great rainstorm broke. He went to take shelter in the den of a jackal in the corner of a cave until the rain stopped. A revelation came to him saying, "Get out of the jackal's den for the jackal's young cannot rest because of you there." Jesus cried aloud, saying, "Lord, the jackal's young have a shelter but the son of Mary has no shelter, no place where he may dwell?"

Yes, the jackal's young have a home but they have no such Beloved to drive them out of their home. Spiritual warriors have such a One driving them out. If they do not own their own home, what does that matter? The loving kindness of such a Driver and the Grace of such a robe of honor that they should have been singled out by God to drive them forth is worth far more than a hundred thousand heavens and earths.

There is a bipolar responsibility involved in this friendship. On the one hand, it is to love God and those who love God reflected in helping God's friends and being enemies of God's enemies including their ego and satanic temptations. Those who manifest this Sign in their relationships with others help their friends to overcome their difficulties, give them guidance, a sense of peace and success in this world. To be friends of God's friends is to believe in what they believe; to do what they do, to reject what they reject, to love the One that they love.

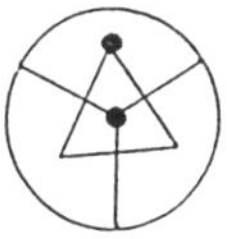

Wisdom

As trustees of nature, spiritual warriors perform the duties that God gave to them in regard to others and overcoming their negative traits. These are signs of the wis dom of the Praiseworthy (al-Ḥamīd). The sign being praiseworthy (*ḥamīd*) is associated with majesty (*jalīl*) and being the highest (*'alī*). Majesty is a sign of the manifestation of the perfection of the qualities and the highest is to remember God and invoke God's qualities.

All of creation praises God with their tongues, their actions, or their very beings in the way they relate to their own species. So, then, should spiritual warriors do the same. "*Nothing there is that does not proclaim His praise*" (17:45). The sunflower in its movement follows the movement of the sun and the selenotrop the movement of the moon, forming a procession within the limits of their power, each singing the praise of the Creator. Each moves to the extent it is free to move and if they could hear the sound of its rotation they would hear a hymn that is within the power of a plant to sing.

Additional Signs of being praiseworthy is when the friends of spiritual warriors praise their beliefs, character, activities, and words because they sing out God's praise, saying, "*al-hamdullāh*," that is, "praise belongs to God," not taking any credit themselves for good they have done to others, for it is God who gave them life, form, strength, intelligence, and speech.

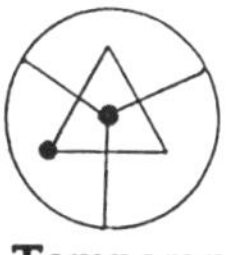

Temperance

In order to add to the trust that they have established with others, spiritual warriors need to be a reckoner (*muḥṣī*) of their relationships manifesting temperance as they analyze their actions and ask their "self' if they are right or wrong according to God's Commands. Through the sign the Reckoner (al-Muḥṣī), the quantity of things are made known. "*Naught there is but its treasuries are with*

Us and We send it not down but in a known measure" (15:21).

When spiritual warriors are hurt by reproaching themselves and are thus made aware of their wrongdoing, that is a proof that God loves them and cares for them. But if the reproach flows over them and does not hurt them, then this is no proof of love. When a carpet is beaten to get rid of the dust, it is not called a reproach but if a parent disciplines his own child, then this is called a reproach and is a proof of love. Therefore so long as they perceive pain and regret within themselves, that is proof that God loves them and cares for them.

If they perceive a fault in their brother, the fault which they perceive in him is within themselves. The learned person is like a mirror in which they see their own image for "the believer is the mirror of his fellow believer." They need to get rid of that fault in themselves for what distresses them in another distresses them in themselves. An elephant was led to a well to drink. Perceiving itself in the water, it shied away. It supposed that it was shying away from another elephant and did not realize that it was from itself that it shied away.

All qualities of oppression, hatred, envy, greed, mercilessness, pride, when they are within themselves do not pain people. When they perceive them in another then they shy away and are pained. People feel no disgust at their own scab and abscess but if they see a tiny abscess or half a scratch on another's hand, they shy away from that person's hand. Wrongdoings are like scabs and abscesses.

Just as they shy away from their brother, so they should excuse him if he shies away from them and is pained. The pain they feel is his excuse because their pain comes from perceiving those faults and he perceives the same faults—"the believer is the mirror of his fellow believer."

Another way of putting it is to see their wrong and corrupt thoughts as thieves who rob them of their capital, that is, their life. These corrupt thoughts develop multiple ways of cunning in order to succeed in corrupting their 'self'. Once spiritual warriors are able to reframe these thoughts, they can turn the thief within into a policeman who acts with benevolence and justice using exactly the same cunning as before but now for the right reasons.

Temperance

The tension between the next two Signs, the Beginner (al-Mubdi') and the Restorer (al-Mu'īd) are Names of the attributes the Constrictor (al-Qābiḍ) and the Expander (al-Bāṣit). Just as spiritual warriors recognize that they are God's trustees on earth, they seek to manifest temperance as they try to understand their origins and the Beginner (al-Mubdi') how they live, grown, see, hear, speak, and think through innate processes that do not necessarily require their consciousness.

Temperance

Finally, consciousness of the trust helps them to understand the secret of the end and restorer (*mu'īd*). In their relationships with others, they may originate a friendship or they may restore a lost one. In either case, whether they are referring to beginnings or ends, there is something put in charge of them which does not allow them to speak. Though that controller is imperceptible to them, yet when they feel yearning and compulsion and pain they know that there is a controller. For instance, they enter the water. The softness of the flowers and fragrant herbs reaches them. When they go to the other side, thorns prick into them. It thus becomes known to them that on that side is a thorn bed and discomfort and pain while on the other side is a flower bed and ease although they perceive neither. This is called emotion and it is more apparent than anything perceptible. For instance, hunger and thirst, anger and happiness—all these things are imperceptible yet they are more apparent than anything perceptible. For if spiritual warriors close their eyes they do not see the perceptible whereas they cannot by any device drive hunger away from themselves. Similarly, hotness in hot dishes and coldness, sweetness and bitterness in foods, these are imperceptible yet they are more apparent than anything perceptible.

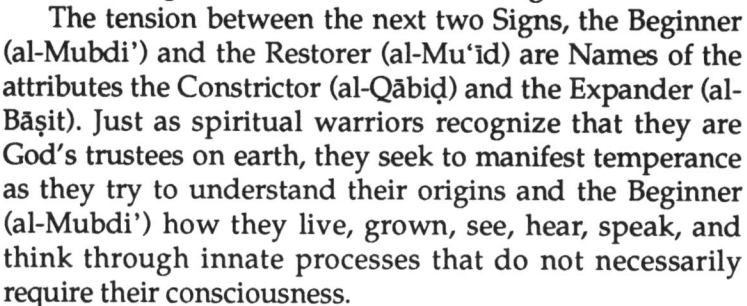

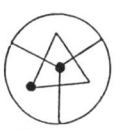

As to their beginning (*mubdi'*), the immediate origins of their physical self are their mothers and fathers who are like bees uniting the seeker with the sought and bringing together the lover and the beloved. They then suddenly fly away. God, however, is the Originator, and He has made their parents a means for uniting the wax and the honey and then they fly away to another part of the garden, but the wax and honey remain and the garden.

As to ends, if a person should sit with a corpse in a tomb even for a moment there is fear that he may go mad. God has appointed that to strike fear into people's hearts and as a token to renew that striking of fear again and again so that a terror may be manifest in the hearts of people because of the desolation of the tomb and the dark earth. In the same way when a caravan has been ambushed in a certain place on the road, two or three stones are placed together there to act as a waysign as much as to say, "Here is a place of danger." These graves are a visible waysign indicating a place of danger.

Some people look at the beginning and some look at the end. These who look at the end are great and mighty people for their gaze is fixed on the issue and the world beyond. But those who look at the beginning are more elect. They say, "What need is there for us to look at the end? If wheat is sown at the beginning, barley will not grow at the end; if barley is sown, wheat will not grow." So their gaze is fixed on the beginning. There are other people still more elect who look neither at the beginning nor at the end, the beginning and the end do not enter their minds. They are absorbed in God. And there are yet other people who are absorbed in worldly things. They look neither at the beginning nor at the end as well, but do so being exceedingly heedless. These are those who have gone astray.

CHAPTER SEVEN

PERFECTING THEIR INSTINCTIVE PERCEPTION THROUGH NOBLE CHARACTER DEVELOPMENT

Strengthening their character, which is formed from their perception of the world and then serves as the basis of their relationships with others, spiritual warriors begin by cleansing their hearts of worldly desires (*muḥyī*), dying to their false self (*mumīt*), and becoming conscious of self (*ḥayy*), detaching their hearts from everything other than God (*qayyūm*). When they are so detached, they have no needs but God (*wajīd*) and manifest a glory and richness of character (*majīd*). They find everything they need to grow closer to God in the perfection of their character which is found in the One (*wāḥid*) whereby they manifest a unity of character (*aḥad*) which is incomparable to everything else whether it be external or internal. Through this refinement of their character, they become models for others (*ṣamad*).

APPLICATION

Working towards refining their character, spiritual warriors bring life to their heart by cleansing it of any worldly desires or attachments at the same time that through hard work for God's sake, they are able to serve His creatures continuously as if they will never die. Recalling paradoxes, they realize, however, that at the same time they continuously remember death and work for their own salvation. Instead, they concentrate, while alive (*muḥyī*), on manifesting temperance in perfecting their faith, acquiring wisdom and prudence and gathering its fruits, and preparing for the Hereafter.

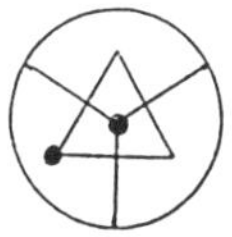

Temperance

Sensing their being alive is to have regard for the means by which they have attained this stage. They may meet up with a fatalist who tells them that nothing can help them against their destiny and that it is useless to stand against the Divine Decree. One answer to such a statement is that the Messenger presents the model of someone who held the means to attaining something important. He said, "Trust in God yet tie the camel's leg." While trusting in God, neglect not the means for "the worker is the friend of God." They need to remember to exert themselves in order to attain their needs bit by bit.

The fatalist may then say, "Whatever the poor gain by their exertions is but a small morsel that will not bring them luck. Self-exertion springs from weakness and to rely on anything but God is a blot upon perfect trust. Certainly self-exertion is not more noble than trust in God." They may continue their argument saying, "What is more beautiful than to commit yourself to God? Many a person has fled from one danger only to be confronted by an even greater one—like fleeing from a snake only to meet up with a dragon. People plan all sorts of strategies and thereby ensnare themselves. What one takes for life ends up being death—shuts the door after his enemy is inside his home. Their eyes are weak in comparison to His. They need no more than His sight. Can He who sends down rain from heaven not provide us with their daily bread?"

In response, those who manifest 'being alive' (*muḥyī*) respond that it is as if He set a ladder before their feet so that step by step they might climb to the roof. Fatalism has no place here. They have feet—why pretend they can't walk? They have hands—why conceal them? Self-exertion is giving thanks for God's blessings. Does fatalism give such thanks? Giving thanks for blessings increases blessings but fatalism snatches those blessings away. If they really have trust in God, they need to exert themselves and feel being alive and strive in constant reliance upon God.

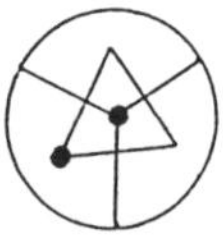
Temperance

Alive through helping others, spiritual warriors can only do that successfully when they die to their own false self (*mumīt*). When they die to their false self (ego), their relations with others become illuminating experiences.

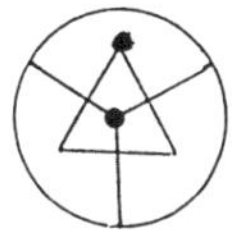
Wisdom

There is a well known Tradition of the Messenger which says, "Die before you die." This refers to dying to one's ego which is one's false identity and being reborn and living (*ḥayy*) through a purified heart.

Rumi tells the story of a mystic who came upon a peacock that was plucking out its feathers. The mystic asked, "Peacock, why are you plucking out such fine feathers from the very root? How can your heart bear you to pluck off these splendid gifts and fling them in the mud. Those who know the Quran by heart so treasure and admire your every feather that they put them between the leaves of the Quran. People make fans of your feathers to stir the air. What ingratitude! What recklessness! Do you not know who painted them? Or are you just showing off by deliberately doing this?"

The peacock answered, "If I were doing this to show off I would cause myself to lose favor with God. Humility is the safe way. I do it out of humility."

"Do not pluck out your feathers," the mystic responded. "Do you not see your own beauty? It is a prerequisite of the greater *jihād* that there should be an enemy to fight. When there is no enemy, there is no *jihād*. If you were without desires, you cannot act according to God's command. Self-control is meaningless if you have no desire. When there is no opponent what need do you have of strength? Do not castrate yourself. Do not become a monk. Chastity is dependent upon desire. Unless desire exists, it is impossible to deny it. What heroism is there in fighting the dead? Do not take the face of contentment out of covetousness. Do not rend the cheek of humility out of arrogance. Do not rend the face of generosity out of greed. Do not pluck out those feathers which are an ornament to Paradise, those feathers which wing you upon the Way."

Just as a fruit fails if it lacks a kernel, so, too, it fails without a skin. If you sow a seed in the earth without its husk, it fails to germinate whereas if you bury it in the earth with its husk, it does germinate and becomes a great tree. So from this point of view of the body, too, is a great and necessary principle and without it, tasks fail and the purpose is not attained.

The animal self is the enemy of spiritual warriors and God's enemy. "*Take not My enemy and your enemy for friends*" (60:1). Spiritual warriors strive always against this enemy while the self is imprisoned in the physical form. When the self is in prison and calamity and pain occurs then deliverance appears and gathers strength. A thousand times it has been proven to them that deliverance comes to them out of toothache and headache and fear. Why then are they chained to physical comfort? Why are they ever occupied with tending the flesh? Forget not the end of the thread: spiritual warriors learn to constantly deny their animal self its desires until they have attained their eternal desire and find deliverance out of the prison of darkness. "*But as for him who feared the Station of his Lord and forbade the soul its caprice, surely Paradise shall be the refuge*" (89:40-41). Being reborn in one's true self is to live through a sense of temperance.

Wisdom

Their character is further strengthened when they are able to attain detachment (*qayyūm*) from everything but God and they meet the needs of others in God's Name, the Self-Existing (al- Qayyūm). A sign that this quality has not been manifest is in those who are heedless and deny the infinite good of creation as they manifest justice.

When the desire to grow closer to God is present at the moment of truth, this desire will act as a veil upon spiritual warriors. So it is with all desires and affections, all loves and fondnesses which people have for every variety of thing—mother, father, heaven, earth, gardens, palaces, branches of knowledge, acts, things to eat and drink. The servant of God realizes that all these desires are the desire for God and all those things are veils. When servants pass out of this world and behold the Creator without these veils, then they will realize that all those were veils and coverings, their quest being in reality that One Thing. All difficulties will then be resolved, and they will hear in their hearts the answer to all questions and all problems

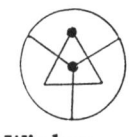

and everything will be seen face to face.

God has created these veils for a good purpose. For if God's beauty should display itself without a veil, they would not have the power to endure and would not enjoy it. Through the intermediary of these veils they derive succor and benefit. You see yonder sun, how in its light they walk and see and distinguish good from bad and are warmed. The trees and orchards become fruitful and in the heat of it, their fruits, unripe and sour and bitter, become mature and sweet. Through its influence mines of gold and silver, rubies and cornelians are made manifest. If the sun, which through intermediaries bestows so many benefits, were to come nearer, it would bestow no benefit whatsoever. On the contrary, the whole world and every creature would be burned up and destroyed. When God makes revelation through a veil to the mountain, it too becomes fully arrayed in trees and flowers and green. When however He makes revelation without a veil, He overthrows the mountain and breaks it into atoms. "*And when his Lord revealed Him to the mountain, He made it crumble into dust*" (7:139). It is then that they have no worldly needs because they lack nothing (*wajīd*) and express wisdom.

Wisdom

There once was a resourceful bird which inadvertently fell into a trap. The bird said to the hunter, "Noble sir, you have eaten many oxen and sheep. You have sacrificed many camels yet you have never been filled by them. Surely you will not become filled by eating my little joints. Permit me to give you three pieces of advice so that you may decide for yourself if I am wise or a fool. From these three counsels you will gain good luck. What I have to say, first of all, is this: Don't believe an absurdity from anyone."

Having given its first weighty piece of advice, the bird broke free and flew upon a wall. "Don't grieve over what is past. That's the second advice," the bird said. "Once something is over and passed beyond your power, don't regret it." Then it said to the hunter, "There is a pearl hid-

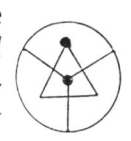

den in my body. It weights ten grams. As sure as you're a living soul, that jewel was your fortune and your children's luck. Now you've missed the pearl since you weren't fated to possess it yet the like of that pearl is not to be found."

The hunter was overcome with grief. The bird said, "Didn't I counsel you well not to grieve over yesterday's past? Since it is past and gone, what's the use of grieving? Either you didn't understand my advice or you're deaf. Then the second piece of advice that I gave you was not to be so misguided as to believe an absurd statement—I don't weigh three grams myself so how could ten grams weight be inside of me?"

The hunter then returned to his senses. "Well, then, tell me your third good counsel," he said.

"A fine use you've made of what I've already told you," said the bird, "that I should tell you the third counsel gratuitously."

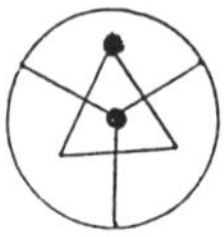

Wisdom

As spiritual warriors, they are given whatever they wish. They then find what God wishes them to find. They manifest their portion of glory (*majīd*) because of their character, manifesting wisdom. God gives them Signs of how to develop good conduct and character so that they are able to do good deeds. Signs that they manifest this quality are gifts from God such as rewards for forgiving their sins and hiding their faults from others. They, in turn, protecting the rights of the rightful, help relieve their difficulties. God then prepares the cause for their peace, happiness, and salvation.

They may be aware of one thing while they are unaware of another. Whereas earth, inanimate as it is, is aware of what God has given it for if it were unaware, how would it have been receptive to water and how would it have nursed and nourished every seed accordingly? When they apply themselves earnestly and attentively to a particular task, their attentiveness to that task means that they are unaware of any other. By this inattention they do not mean total inattention—some people

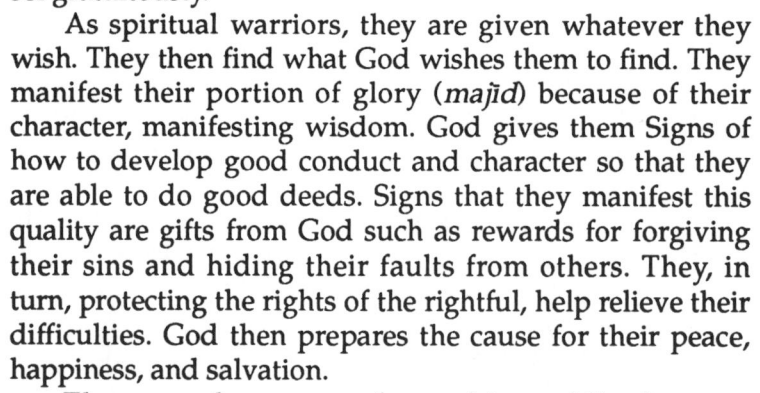

wanted to catch a cat but found it impossible to do so. One day that cat was preoccupied with hunting a bird and became inattentive through hunting the bird so they caught it.

In order to manifest good character and conduct, it is not necessary to become totally preoccupied with worldly affairs. They must take them easily and not be in bondage to them. Otherwise, no matter what they do, someone will always be dissatisfied with them. When this effects them, they are no longer able to transform themselves. If for instance they have many kinds of cloth of every sort, when they are absorbed, why, which of them will they clutch? Though all are indispensable, yet it is certain that in the bundle they will lay hands on something precious and to be treasured for with one pearl and a single ruby one can make a thousand decorations.

From a certain tree sweet fruit materializes though that fruit is a part of it yet God has chosen and distinguished that part above the whole for in it. He deposited a sweetness that He did not deposit in the rest and by virtue of that, that part become superior to that whole and proved the purpose of the tree.

In furthering their expression of good character and conduct within themselves, it helps them to strip their discriminative faculty of all prejudices and to seek a friend in the faith. Faith consists in knowing who is one's true friend. When, however, they have spent their life in the company of people who lack discrimination, their own discriminative faculty becomes feeble and they are unable to recognize that true friend of the faith because they have nurtured a friendship in which there is no discernment. Discernment is that one quality which is hidden in a person. They see that a madman possesses hands and feet but lacks discernment? Discernment is that subtle essence which is within them. Day and night they have been occupied with nurturing that physical substance without discernment. They put forward as a pretext that that subsists through this. Yet this likewise subsists through that. How is it that they have devoted all their energies to looking after the physical substance and have entirely neglected the subtle essence? Indeed, the physical subsists through the other whereas the other is by no means dependent upon the physical for its subsistence.

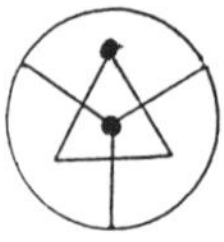

Wisdom

At this stage, they manifest perfection of character (*wāḥīd*) in being unique as they relate to others. Their relationships are such that they can neither be divided nor duplicated. Signs of the manifestation of this quality are good character, good morals, and manners. The secret of this sign is to understand the unity in all of the Signs. And then they attain to the oneness of self (*aḥad*) which unites all qualities and manifests unity in multiplicity (uniqueness) and multiplicity in unity (oneness).

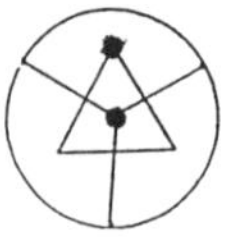

Wisdom

Anṣarī says, "To know One refers to service, conduct, and resolution. In service, it means to forego leadership, observe sincerity, and control thought. In conduct, it means to purify the inmost consciousness, actualize remembrance, and cling steadily to confidence. In resolution, it means to lose and to forget everything but God and to be delivered through the heart's freedom from all other than He."

When spiritual warriors are able to actually assume these traits, they forget the qualities that others attribute to them or they yourselves think that they have so that they see the self as a single identity and sense a oneness in their relationships with others so that each 'I' becomes 'they'. This gives a quality of incomparability whereby no person or relationship can be compared to them within or without. It is then that they manifest uniqueness.

> Say not two, know not two, call not on two!
> Know the slave is obliterated in his lord!
> So the lord is obliterated in God that created him;
> Yea, lost and dead and buried in his Creator!
> When you regard this lord as separate from God,
> You annihilate at once text and paraphrase.
> With eyes and heart look beyond mere water and
> clay,

God alone is the Qiblah; regard not two Qiblahs!
If you regard two, you lose the benefit of both;
A spark falls on the tinder and the tinder vanishes.

In regard to unity Aṭṭār says:

Come you lost atoms,
to your center draw
And be the Eternal Mirror
that you saw
Rays that have wandered
into darkness wide
Return and back
into your Sun subside [1]

When the wind blows through a house it lifts up the edge of the carpet and the rugs all flap and move about. It whisks into the air sticks and straws, ruffles the surface of the pool until it looks like a coat of chain mail, sets trees and twigs and leaves a-dancing. All those states appear distinct and different, but from the standpoint of the object and root and reality, they are one thing only inasmuch as they are all set in motion by the one wind. This is explained by Rūmī when he ways:

I died from mineral and plant became;
Died from the plant and took a sentient frame;
Died from the beast and donned a human dress.
When by my dying did I ever grow less?
Another time from humanhood I must die
To soar with angel-pinions through the sky.
Amidst angels also I must lose my place
Since '*Everything shall perish save His Face (Presence).*'
Let me be naught! the harp-strings tell me plain
That unto Him do we return again!

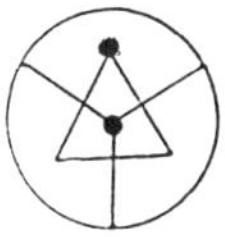
Wisdom

Finally, at this stage, if they have received the blessings of God, they should be able to be a model for others (*ṣamad*) by sensing a religious duty to educate God's creation, satisfying their needs, and showing them, through their words and actions, God's way to fulfilling their worldly and religious duties as they manifest wisdom and prudence. The manifestation of this Sign, however, is not to just meet the needs of others but to satisfy the needs of others the way they should be satisfied and not necessarily as they want.

Substance is like a musk-pod and this material world and its delights are like the scent of the musk. The scent of the musk is but transient for it is mere accident. If spiritual warriors seek the scent of the musk itself and be not content with only the scent, they gain goodness. But they who have been satisfied to possess the scent are wronged for they have grasped after a thing that does not remain in their hand. For the scent is merely the attribute of the musk. So long as the musk is apparent in this world, its scent comes to the nostrils. When however it enters the veil and returns to the other world, all those who lived by its scent die. For the scent is attached to the musk and departs whereas the musk reveals itself.

Happy are they who reach the musk through the scent and become one with the musk. Thereafter there remains no passing away for them; they have become eternal in the very essence of the musk and take on the predicament of the musk. Thereafter they communicate its scent to the world and the world is revived by them. Only the name of what they were survives in them as with a horse or any other animal that has turned to salt in a salt-pan, only the name of horse remains to it. In effect and influence it is that ocean of salt. What harm does that name do to it? It will not bring it out of its saltiness. And if they give some other name to this salt-mine, it will not lose its saltiness.

So it behooves spiritual warriors to seek these pleasures and delights which are the ray and reflection of God. They must not become content with this much even though this much is of God's Grace and the radiance of His beauty, yet it is not eternal. With reference to God, He is eternal. With reference to the human being, their body is not everlasting. It is like the rays of the sun which shine into a house for all that they are the rays of the sun and are light, yet they are attached to the sun. When the sun sets, the light no more remains. Hence it behooves spiritual warriors to become the sun so that the fear of separation may no more remain.

CHAPTER EIGHT

PERFECTING THEIR INSTINCTIVE MOTIVATION THROUGH NOBLE ACTIONS

In perfecting their actions and directing their motivations towards assuming the noble character traits in their relations with others, spiritual warriors realize they are able (*qadīr*) and powerful (*muqtadir*). They pray to be advanced (*muqaddim*) on the path and not to have it postponed (*mu'akhkhir*) because of their actions or weakness of motivation. They take the initiative and become first (*awwal*) in their devotions among their friends and the last (*ākhir*) to reproach them for their negative traits. They manifest (*ẓāhir*) perfection of their potential true self, hidden (*bāṭin*) within themselves. They act towards others as a governor (*wālī*), controlling their 'self' from rebelling against God's commands. They confess their belief in God (*muta'ālī*), doing good (*barr*) to others, being a repenter (*tawwāb*) of their past mistakes and being an avenger (*muntaqim*) towards their enemies within which prevents them from forming friendships of perfect harmony and unique beauty. They erase (*'afū*) the wrongdoings others have done to them as the final step in perfecting their actions and motivations.

APPLICATION

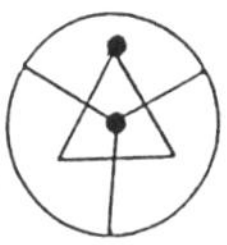

Wisdom

Spiritual warriors manifested spiritual power at the fifth stage with the understanding of being majestic (*jalīl*). When they express being able (*qadīr*), they manifest wisdom by perfecting their actions, directing their motivations, empowering their 'self' with a power which has been defined by Algazel as "the intention by which a thing comes into existence according to a determinate plan of will and knowledge and in conformity with both of them." Spiritual warriors cause things to happen through their will power because their will power is one with God's Will. Creation is often defined as a mirror in which God's Will is reflected.

A Sultan held a competition between Greek and Chinese artists to determine who were the better artists. They were each given a room to display their talents. The two rooms faced each other, the doors of one opening onto the doors of the other. The Chinese took one and the Greeks took the other. The Chinese asked for hundreds of different colors of paint. The Greeks asked for none having planned among themselves to clear the walls of rust. Each shut their doors to the other and worked diligently.

When the Chinese had completed their work, they began to drum for joy. The Sultan went and saw their paintings. The moment he saw them, he was exhilarated from the beauty and splendor of their art. He then moved to the room which displayed the talent of the Greeks. The Greeks removed the curtain so that the reflection of the Chinese masterpieces struck upon the walls they had scoured clean of rust so that it mirrored the work of the Chinese. All that the Sultan had seen in the Chinese room showed lovelier here because instead of trying to imitate the work of the Creator, the Greeks were able to reflect His work. The Sultan's eyes were overwhelmed.

The heart of the one moving closer to God is also like a mirror. Purifying it of greed and covetousness, avarice and malice is, in effect, to remove the rust from the mirror surface and to return to its original purity. It is then that the heart is able to reflect the innumerable images. Every new image that enters the heart shows forth within it free of all imperfection. Those who have polished the surface of their hearts have escaped from attachment to scent or color. At every moment they instantly behold beauty.

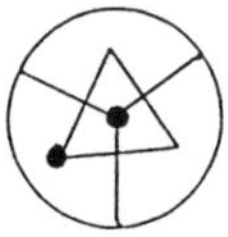

Temperance

When they manifest a more emphatic sign of power and perfecting of their actions and motivations, they express being powerful (*muqtadir*) through temperance. Perfecting their actions and motivations, they empower themselves to some extent but Real power comes from

God Who is the source of all power. They who submit to God's Will receive far greater energies than when they fight it or rebel against it and try to survive on their own very limited power.

When Hannah gave birth to Mary, she vowed to God to dedicate her to the House of God and not to do anything for her. She left her in a corner of the Temple. Zachariah demanded to look after the child. Everyone requested to do the same. A dispute arose between them. Now in that time it was the custom that each party to a dispute should throw a stick into water; the one whose stick floated was deemed to prevail. It so happened that Zachariah's lot was the right one. They said, "He has the right." So every day Zachariah brought food to the child and always found the very match of it in the corner of the temple. He said, "Mary, after all I am in charge of you. Where do you get this?" Mary said, "Whenever I feel the need of food, whatever I request, God sends to me. His bounty and compassion are infinite; whosoever relies on Him, his trust is not in vain." Zachariah said, "Oh, God, since You give every person his need, I also have a desire. Grant me a son who shall be Your friend, who without my prompting shall consort with You and be occupied with obedience to You." God brought John the Baptist into being after his father was bent and feeble and his mother, too, who had not borne any child while she had been young, being now of great age again had her course and became pregnant.

Signs of those who perfect their actions and motivations are God's gifts of ease, wisdom, patience, perseverance, and strength. This power or spiritual energy is expressed after having submitted to God's Will, obeying God's Will, loving and fearing God. Once this force or energy is in place, nothing can overcome it.

Prayer is a means to attain to this power. By prayer it is not meant that they should be standing and bowing and prostrating all day. Its purpose is that it is necessary that that spiritual state which possesses spiritual warriors visibly when they are at prayer should be with them always. Whether sleeping or waking, whether writing or reading, in all circumstances they should not be free from God's hand so that "*They continue at their prayer,*" (70:23) will apply also to them. Speaking and remaining silent, sleeping and eating, being enraged and forgiving—all those attributes are the turning of a water-mill which revolves. Undoubtedly this revolving of the mill is by means of the water because it has made trial of itself also without any water. So if the water-mill considers that turning to proceed from itself, that is the very acme of foolishness and ignorance. This revolving takes place within a narrow space. Cry unto God saying, "Oh God, grant to me, instead of my present journey and revolving, another revolving which shall be spiritual; seeing that all needs are fulfilled by You and Your bounty and compassion are universal over all creatures."

In order to perfect their actions, they need to constantly be in a state of remembrance of Him. For the remembrance of Him is strength and feathers and wings to the bird of the spirit. If that purpose is wholly realized, that is "*Light upon Light,*" (24:35). By the remembrance of God, little by little the inward heart becomes illumined and detachment from the world is realized. For instance, just as a bird desires to fly into heaven, although it does not reach the heaven, yet every moment it rises farther from the earth and out soars the other birds. Or, for instance, some musk is in a box and the lid of the box is narrow. They insert their hand into the box but cannot extract the musk, yet for all that their hand becomes perfumed and their nostrils are gratified. So too is the remembrance of God: though they do not attain the Essence of God, yet the remembrance of God leaves its mark on them and great benefits are procured from the recollection of Him.

All naturally love those who love God and those who fear God. There are dangers, however, in this strength which manifest themselves as self-confidence instead of a sense of humility. To maintain the Sign, spiritual warriors needs to remain thankful to God, to repent for mistakes made, to be just, forgiving, generous, and compassionate even to one's enemies. Signs of those who do not manifest power and who rebel against joining God's Will are heedlessness, ambition, seeking of pleasures, self-centeredness and egotism.

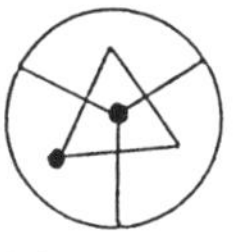

Temperance

In perfecting their actions, they strengthen their sense of temperance by praying to be advanced (*muqaddim*) on the path. The Promoter (al-Muqaddim) is the Sign of manifesting the attributes of action and motivating others to grow close to God, controlling those who are going to advance and those who have moved ahead in order to attain a closeness to God in their relations with others. This closeness comes through worship and doing things to please God. It is to use their actions in their relations with others which are in harmony with His Will. Some advance and some regress. When they manifest the Sign the Promoter (al-Muqaddim), they try to alter the motives of those who rebel and are manifesting al-Mu'akhkhir through a sign of temperance. In a Divine Tradition (*ḥadith qudsī*), God says, "The believer remains eager to meet Me, but I am more eager to meet the believer," and "I advance one cubit for one who advances to Me half a cubit." They help those who rebel against the God's Law, who go astray, who tyrannize themselves and others by helping to postpone their punishment until they can change.

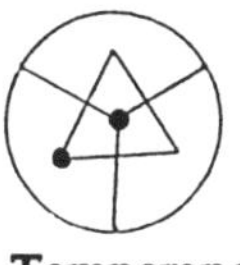

Temperance

When spiritual warriors become conscious of regressing, they need to search for the reason for it. Perhaps they have some impurity of heart remaining or perhaps they are manifesting hypocrisy in their intentions. They need to strive harder. Perhaps God is testing them with a more difficult test or to see the limit of the pain that they can bear. This is why so many pray that God not test them to their limit.

While spiritual warriors persist in wrongdoing and stubbornly refuse to see their errors, why are they so proud that God treats them with patience, kindness, and generosity in spite of their wrongdoings? Is it that they are fooled by what the devil whispers in their ear, saying, "If it were not for your wrongdoings and your revolt, how would God manifest His infinite mercy, compassion, and generosity?" Do you not see how irrational that evil teaching is? Would it be less merciful and beneficent for the Owner of Infinite Wisdom to prevent His servant from opposing His Will and pleasure?

Then the devil may whisper in their ear again: "You have no hope of attaining the level of benevolence of those who are born with good character and obedience. They have come to this world and shown their obedience to the Will of God, gathered their Lord's mercy and beneficence in this world, and left it. The real mercy, generosity and kindness of God will be manifest in the Hereafter on the Day of Judgment when He judges His disobedient servants who are in need of His mercy."

Only those who have lost their senses could believe in and be deceived by such thoughts. They need to protect themselves against such temptations and tell their ego, "What you say about God's infinite patience and generosity towards His servants is true. Indeed, if there were no revolt and disobedience, they would not see the manifestation of His Divine Attributes. So many examples are related in the holy books and statements. But you, evil one, are using the truth for your own purposes—so that God's mercy be manifest, you encourage me to wrongdoing! You are trying to make me revolt because God is patient and kind. You ask me to test God's mercy and beneficence. How do you know, O accursed one, that I am of those who will be forgiven? Indeed God forgives whom He Wills and punishes in justice whom He Wills. How do I know to which party I belong? All I know is that I am full of wrongdoing. And just as I was left in this world without the ability to repent and ask His forgiveness, He may well refuse me His mercy before I enter hell and punish me with the fire. Although one dies as one lives, and wrongdoing is the messenger of disbelief, if I am fortunate and give my last breath as a believer, then He will purify me in hellfire and take me out and give me peace in His mercy.

"If I knew for sure that there were no day of reckoning with my wrongdoing, that there were no punishment and if I were certain that I would receive divine absolution, I might have considered your twisted reasoning. Even then, it would be no better than admitting foolishness for it is certainly an unforgivable behavior for a servant to test the patience of His Lord.

"On the other hand, even if I were certain that I would receive divine punishment, the proper thing for me would be shame and thankfulness for His delaying His punishment and spending of the effort of which I am capable in trying to obey the commands of my Lord.

" I have not heard of any good word that all wrongdoing will be forgiven. On the contrary, one is left free to choose between the positive and the negative, and the Ultimate Judge is free to forgive or to punish. In your case, though, O evil-commanding ego, there is no choice. You are constant in your wish for the wrong and the forbidden!"

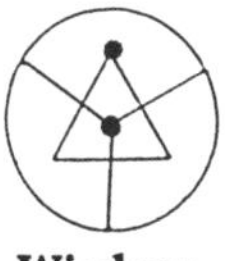

Wisdom

Expressions of the Signs the First (al-Awwal), the Last (al-Ākhir), the Manifest (al-Ẓāhir) and the Hidden (al-Batin) known as the "mother of the noble character traits," take the form of being just and fair in their relations with others. To be first in positive deeds towards others and last to reproach others for their negative traits, is to improve their actions and strengthen their motivations to the positive. They practice meeting a kindness with a greater kindness and an offense with something less.

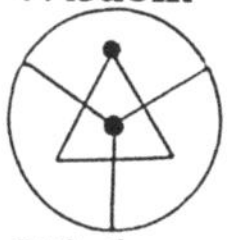

Wisdom

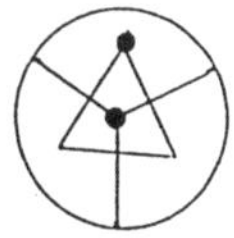

Wisdom

The wisdom of the actions of spiritual warriors towards others becomes manifest when their actions in their relations to others are orderly because the self can only be seen through its effects. At the same time that the self is hidden within, it is the self alone which is constant and is manifest through their actions and their evaluation of the quality of their actions. From another perspective,

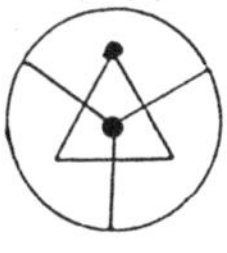

Wisdom

the order that they sense in the universe which they try to manifest in their relations with others is hidden from their senses but apparent or manifest to their reasoning capacity through deduction of its effects.

Expressing their self in its hidden aspect, spiritual warriors invite others to spiritual perfection if they have purified their inner self and if God has bestowed upon them knowledge of the heart. Developing their sense of justice, they manifest a sincere love towards others through which they are inwardly impelled to concern themselves with whatever means necessary to relieve a friend and bestow on him or her whatever is possible. Adam manifest this when he was taught the meaning of the Names. His perfection of faith was thereby made greater.

Angels were told to prostrate themselves before him because the angels only know the manifest, while the human being knows the meaning that the Names contain, the hidden. Expressing their inner or hidden self in its perfection is to follow the Law that God made manifest.

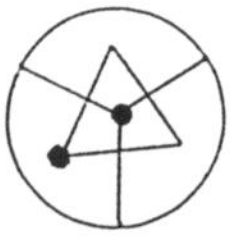

Temperance

The servants who manifest their portion of being a governor (*wālī*) in their relations to others, showing temperance, govern or rule over those entrusted to them according to God's Command. That is, they deal with them through goodness in an organized manifestation of power and action, planning, realizing their plans, and protecting and preserving their plans. These qualities they have developed by using their free will to make God's choice. In this way they help realize, receive, and benefit from what God has written for them. It means understanding that they are free to open their eyes and receive the light of faith and knowledge or to rebel, closing their eyes and remaining in the darkness of ignorance. When they revolt with their free will, whatever is destined to happen to them will still happen but they will be unaware, unconscious, resentful and in a state of disharmony with things around them.

Continuing to perfect their actions through enhancing

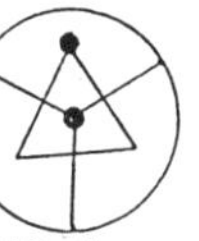

Wisdom

their motivation to seek closeness to God through justice, they attain their portion of the sign al-Muta'ālī which is the intense form of al-'Alī. It is to learn to say, "I believe in God," (*amintu billāhī*). This belief is characterized as the belief in God and God's Most Beautiful Names, moving level by level or stage by stage in understanding God's Signs within and without, remaining in a constant stage of consciousness of, remembrance of, and devotion to God. The goal for their intentions, efforts, and consciousness is knowing, seeking, finding, and being close to God. It is to repeat the prayer taught to the Messenger in the Quran, "*Say: My Lord, increase me in knowledge*" (20:114).

Rightness and goodness of action depends on two bases: fear of God and sincerity of intention or purity of purpose. Fear of God leads to piety (*taqwā*) and this results in greater effectiveness of deeds. Every act, positive or negative, has an effect upon the self. When the act is that of devotion and worship, the effect is to make the physical faculties subservient to the intellectual faculties. As a result, physical nature is made subject to spirituality until the self reaches the stage of spiritual emotion and attains its essential goal. Every act that increases this effect and discharges this service in a better way is more rightful and more effective in attaining the essential goal. The Messenger said, "The best of deeds is the most difficult of them." Thus devotional rites are to tame the corporeal nature and strengthen the self's active will power. Piety, besides being one of the reforming agents of the self, also affects the influence of inward and outward human actions and is the cause of their acceptability. "*Verily God accepts only from the pious*" (5:27).

The second is sincere intention. Nothing is as important in worship as intention for the relationship of intention to worship is like that of the self to the body. In the same way as the physical form originates in the physical aspect of the self, intention and its spirit originates from the self's inward aspect and the heart.

Becoming a doer of good among human beings is to

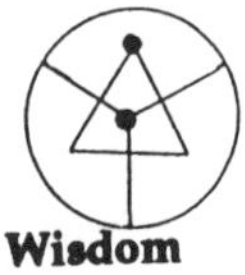

Wisdom

manifest a portion of the Sign the Source of All Goodness (al-Barr). Servants manifest material and spiritual good wishing to do good to all believers because they have immersed themselves in the sea of the mystery of goodness. It is manifest particularly when spiritual warriors do good to parents, teachers, and elders. When they do good to God's creation, they see the reflection of God the Source of All Goodness in themselves. When Prophet Moses talked to his Lord on Mt. Tur, he saw a man standing on the highest point of God's throne. He asked, "Oh Lord, how did this servant reach such heights?" God answered, "He was never envious of the good that I bestowed upon my servants and he was especially good to his mother and father." That is, this servant who attained the highest point manifested a sense of wisdom whereby he controls his irrational aspects of self and relinquishes attempts to control those around him.

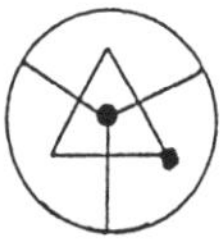

Courage

When through their actions they help others to repent by showing them God's signs, giving counsel to them, and disclosing His warnings to them—the need to know the dangers of their wrongdoings—spiritual warriors may perhaps gain the fear necessary to repent. Turning to God, they become a repenter (*tawwāb*).

The Sign comes from the word *tawbah,* to repent and return to the Straight Path. It is to move from unconsciousness and imbalance to harmony with God's' Will. When accepted, God's anger is transformed into mercy, compassion, and love. When the errors are deeply embedded, they have to dig out the roots or causes for their wrongdoing in order to renounce them. A Sign of the manifestation of a portion of the Repenter (al-Tawwāb) within is when spiritual warriors continue to forgive those who hurt them, never doubting the mercy of God and God's acceptance of sincere repentance manifesting courage. When they repent from inappropriate desires, lying to others, and allowing their imagination to rule their relationships, they come to know the multiplicity of self and achieve unity and oneness.

One day a mule, stabled with a camel, began to complain of his state. "I am often falling on my face. It's the same whether I am on a hill or high-road, in the bazaar or on the street but especially when I am descending from the mountain top. Sheer terror tumbles me down all the time. You, my camel friend, on the other hand, never fall on your face. What's the reason for this? Perhaps your pure soul was destined to be fortunate. Every moment I bruise my knees and bloody my nose because of my fall. I get a beating all the time from the muleteer. It's like a brainless fellow who continuously breaks his vows of repentance. Due to his feeble resolution, he becomes a plaything of his false self. Because he continues to break his vow of repentance, he is beaten over the head from the unseen. He repents again but with languid resolute. Weakness multiplied by weakness! Yet his arrogance is such that he looks with contempt on those who have attained to God. You, oh camel, are a model of a true believer. You never fall on your face and never turn up your nose. What have you got to never stumble, to never all on your face? May I join up with you?"

The camel replied, "You have made amends because you have confessed in my presence. The wrongdoing that you did was not part of your disposition for from original rebellion comes nothing but denial as was the case with Iblis. Adam's lapse was but passing for he repented at once. You have clutched felicity and flung yourself into eternal fortune."

Courage

Though the perfection of their actions during this phase of their journey closer to God, showing courage, any revenge (*muntaqim*) spiritual warriors take against God's enemies is praiseworthy (al-Muntaqim), the worst enemies being their ego and satanic temptations. When ruled by them, they need to take revenge against their idol/ego for wrongdoing or by falling short in their devotions to Him. Bayazid Bistāmī said, "One night I was too lazy to perform certain prayers. I punished myself by depriving myself of water for one year."

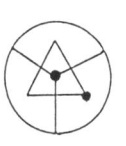

Persistence of errors or wrongdoing come from unconsciousness and egotism resulting in a state of imbalance and tyranny in their relations to others. God warns them, accepts their excuses, delays their punishment in forgiving their sins, but further sin means harder punishment because, as spiritual warriors know, those who serve their own ego instead of becoming God's servant are risking a greater fall. They have been spoiled by God's mercy increasing their arrogance towards others.

Jesus, peace be upon him, was asked, "What is the greatest and most difficult thing in this world and the next?" He replied, "The wrath of God." They asked, "And what shall save a person from that?" He answered, "That you master your own wrath and suppress your rage." Enmity and rage are hidden in their unconsciousness. It is as if they see a spark and a leaping fire which they have to extinguish—"*repel the evil with that which is fairer*" (23:96). They may triumph over their enemies in two ways. First of all, the problem may be with their own thoughts and the person may not be an enemy at all. If so and they can repel the thought from their mind, they repel enmity towards the person, as well.

The second way is for spiritual warriors to adopt a positive attitude toward him even if he be an enemy because this will show up his negative reflections about them. It will become clear that he is not what the person thought he was and that the other person should be reproached and not them. By praising the person and giving thanks to him, they are administering a poison, as it were, for while he is claiming a deficiency in them, they are showing their perfection as the beloved of God Who says, "*... and pardon the offenses of their fellow human beings and God loves the good-doers*" (3:128).

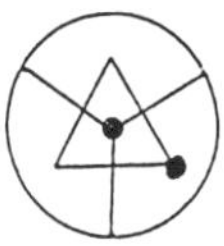

Courage

God's compassion to the believers continues as they seek to perfect their actions or behavior. Seeking to manifest their portion of the Pardoner (al-'Afū) in their relations with others through manifesting courage, knowing that God treats His servants the way they treat others, is to erase and efface wrongdoing done to them by others. They manifest this sign in their relations to others by forgiving those who harm them and, instead, doing good to them. If they relent, their wrongdoings will be erased.

There was a preacher who, whenever he mounted the pulpit, would begin to offer up a prayer for highway robbers. "Lord," he would cry, lifting up his hands, "visit with compassion the wicked, those who do corruption, the insolent wrongdoers, all who make mock of the righteous, all who are infidels at heart, all who dwell in wrongdoing."

He would not say one prayer for the pure. His prayers were always for the depraved. "Such conduct is certainly unusual," people protested. "It is hardly generous to pray for erring people."

"Such are the sorts of people from whom I have derived most good," he answered. "That is why I have singled them out for my prayers. They have treated me with such depravity, oppression, and injustice that they have inadvertently flung me out of wrongdoing into good doing. Every time I turned my face towards this lower material world, they would receive me with blows so I would take refuge from their beatings on the other side. It was the wolves who always brought me back to the right road. Since they contrived the means of my salvation, it is incumbent on me, my clever friends, to pray for them." In other words, every enemy they have is in reality their cure, their sovereign alchemy, their benefactor, their well-wisher.

Chapter Nine
Moving Towards Servanthood by Serving God's Creation

Attaining to the stage of servanthood (*'ubudiyat*) is to have become one with God's Will by disciplining the idol or ego and giving birth to the real self. The stages consist of developing an intense sense of mercy towards others (*ra'ūf*), witnessing God's power (*mālik al-mulk*), finding certainty of faith in the oneness of God (*dhu 'l-jalāl wa 'l-ikrām*), demanding justice for others (*muqsiṭ*), uniting all oppositions through perfect knowledge and proper behavior (*jāmi'*), becoming the servant of God (*ghanī*), with all the material and spiritual richness of servanthood (*mughnī*), avoiding harm and negative influences in their relationships with others (*māni'*) while recognizing that they grow and their educated through pain (*ḍārr*) and understand the operation of God's will in the universe (*nāfi'*).

Application

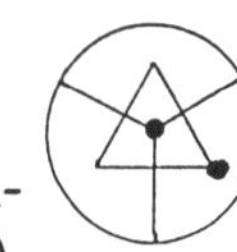
Courage

The Signs of the manifestation of the Clement (al-Ra'uf), an intense form of the Compassionate (al- Raḥīm), in spiritual warriors' relations with others is to show courage and to remember their wrongdoings, to realize God's blessings in spite of their wrongdoings, to try to serve God's creation with both its spiritual and material blessings, to manifest mercy and compassion towards others, and to be clement in everything except when it comes to the punishment required by the God's Law. Although justice as manifested through the Law at times seems harsh, it is a mercy in disguise because through suffering that punishment, their wrongdoings have been paid for in full and will not be put into the balance on the Day of Judgment.

In battling for the faith, the fourth Rightly-Guided

Caliph, 'Alī, overcame a enemy soldier. He quickly drew his sword and made haste to slay him. Thereupon that man spat in 'Alī's face. 'Alī immediately put his sword aside and relaxed his vigor in fighting. The enemy champion was amazed by this deed, by 'Alī's show of clemency and mercy without any apparent reason. He asked him what happened that 'Alī spared his life. 'Alī replied, "It is for God's sake that I wield the sword. When you spat on me, I realized I would be slaying you out of my own anger and not for the sake of God. This I could not do." The sword of clemency is sharper than the sword of steel. Nay, it wins more victories than a hundred hosts.

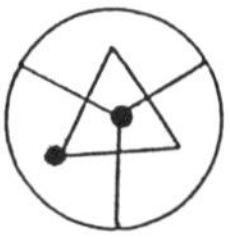

Temperance

Moving forward towards servanthood, spiritual warriors witness God's power (Malik al-Mulk) in the creation becoming God's deputy in governing their relations with others while strengthening their sense of temperance. It is to carry out what God Wills, how God Wills, as God Wills in their relationships.

A certain king flew into a rage with his companion and was on the point of striking him with his sword when one of his courtiers interceded. He did this by prostrating himself on the floor. Seeing this, the king put his sword aside. The king then forgave his companion because of the courtier's intercession, saying to the courtier, "Since you have stepped in between, I am content even though the criminal has done harm a hundredfold. I am able to shatter a hundred thousand rages, seeing that you possess such excellence and worth but your entreaty I cannot in any way shatter since your entreaty is assuredly my own. I had been at the point that indeed if earth and heaven had been dashed together, that man would not have escaped my vengeance. Had every separate atom turned to entreaty, he would not have saved his head from my sword." The king continued, "It was not you noble sir who interceded but truly myself, your attributes being all buried in mine. In this matter you were employed, you were not the prime agent. You are my predicate, not the subject. You enacted God's words, '*When you threw, it was not yourself that threw*' (8:17). You have yielded yourself like foam in the wave. It was not you who gave what you gave, but the King gave. He only is."

The companion, however, having escaped with his life took offense against the intercessor. He severed all bonds of friendship with that true well-wisher, turned his face to the wall, and did not return his greetings. People were astonished. Finally someone asked him, "Why are your treating a well-wisher so unjustly? Your special friend redeemed your life. He saved you from instant execution. Even if he had done you evil, you ought not to shun him. As it was, that admirable friend was your special benefactor."

The man replied, "Why should he intervene as an intercessor? I desire no mercy but the stroke of the King. I desire no refuge except the King. I have naughted all other than the King because I have turned my devotion only to the King. Should the King in his wrath strike off my head, yet He will bestow on me sixty other lives. My business is to stake my head and to be utterly selfless. My King's business is to give me a new head!"

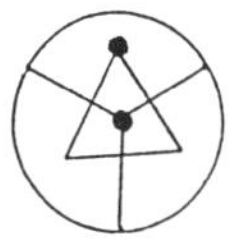
Wisdom

God's generosity and bounty is limitless. God ties us to each other through their needs, both worldly and other worldly. Those who manifest a portion of the Sign of the Lord of Majesty and Generosity (Dhū 'l-Jalāl wa-'l-Ikrām) expect nothing from human beings nor do they fear their condemnation. God is sufficient for them. They should quickly disregard the kingdom of this world like the king, Ibrahim ibn Adham, so that they may attain the kingdom of life everlasting by manifesting a sense of justice in its aspect of fidelity to the Straight Path and putting everything in its proper place.

Nightly Ibrahim ibn Adham was reclining on his throne, busied with the affairs of state, while the palace guards were upon the roof. The king did not intend for his guards to ward off robbers for he knew well that the just man is free from sudden assaults. Secure in his heart, he believed justice would guard him against the wrongdoings of others, not body guards on his roof.

The king spent long evenings listening to the lute like all passionate lovers of God in order to catch, perchance, the faint echo of the Divine rhythm in nature because the plaintive sounds of the lute coupled with the beating of the drum somehow resembled the music of the spheres. Philosophers over the ages have pointed out that they derive these harmonies from the rotation of the heavenly spheres and that those who accompany these instruments with song are but the murmur of the revolving spheres. True believers even say that the influence of Paradise has converted every ugly sound into one of beauty for they are all parts of Adam. They have heard these melodies before although the water and clay from which they were made have cast doubt into their hearts.

One night the king heard a scurry of feet and a commotion on the roof. "Who dares to disturb their peace?" he asked himself. "Who is there?" he shouted at the palace windows. "This cannot be of human kind. It must be of the *jinn*."

A strange folk put down their heads from the room. He asked, "What are you seeking?"

"Camels," they replied.

"Camels?" echoed the king. "Who ever sought camels on a roof?"

"Then how," they demanded of him, "do you seek to meet God seated on your throne of pomp?"

That sufficed. No man ever saw the king again. He vanished from humanity as though he were a *jinn*.

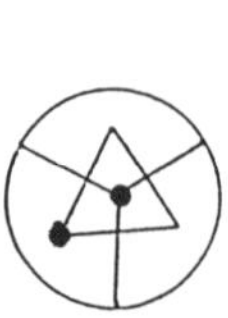

Temperance

Spiritual warriors develop a perfect sense of measure seeing things in a fair and just way. From this they come to demand justice for others but not for themselves. They learn to protect those who should be protected and help those who should be helped (*muqsiṭ*) as they manifest temperance. There is a famous hadith in this regard, Caliph 'Umar asked the Messenger why he was smiling. The Messenger said, "I see two men among my people who are before God. One says, 'Oh Lord, take from this man that which is rightfully mine!' God tells the other man, 'Give to your brother what belongs to him.' The usurper responds, 'Oh Lord, I have no good deeds with which to repay this man.' God turns to the wronged one and says, 'What should I do to your brother? He has nothing left to give you.' The wronged one says, 'Oh Lord, let him take some of my wrongdoings.'

"At this point, tears welled up in the Messenger's eyes and he said, 'That day is the Day of Judgment. That day is the day when each person will wish others to carry his wrongdoings.' Then he continued, 'After the wronged one has wished the usurper to take over some of his wrongdoings, God asks him to lift his head and look at Paradise.'

"He says, 'Oh Lord, I see cities of silver and palaces of gold bedecked with pearls. For which Prophet, which saint, which martyr are these palaces?'

"God says, 'The are for those who can pay their price.'

"The man who had been wronged says, 'Who could possibly pay the prices of these?'

"God said, 'Perhaps you could.' The man says, 'How, oh Lord? I have nothing. What could I do to gain the price of Paradise?'

"God the Equitable (al-Muqsiṭ) says, 'By forgiving your brother, by giving up your claim in that which he took from you.'

"The wronged man says, 'I forgive him, my Lord. I do not want my right.' All the Merciful, the Generous says, 'Then hold your brother's hand and enter My Paradise together.'"

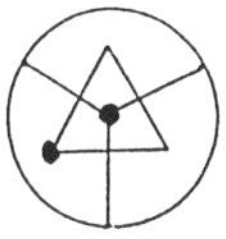

Temperance

At this point, moving towards servanthood as spiritual warriors manifest wisdom in caring for their relatives, they are able to gather together (*jāmi'*) their external behavior towards others and the truths hidden in their heart. Perfect knowledge of these truths results in proper behavior towards others. The light of knowledge of those who manifest this Sign does not diminish their sense of humility towards others because their knowledge is combined with self-restraint and insight. They are able to unite what which is dissimilar, different, and opposites both within and without. Through the manifestation of the sign the Gatherer (al-Jāmi') they are able to gather and manifest the Most Beautiful Names in this stage of perfecting servanthood.

Rūmī tells us, "Do they not see how the spring breeze becomes visible in the trees and grasses, the rose-beds and sweet herbs? Through the medium of these they gaze upon the beauty of spring. But when they look upon the spring breeze itself, they see nothing of these things. It is not because those spectacles and rosebeds are not in the breeze; after all, are these not its rays? Rather, within the spring breeze are waves of rosebeds and sweet herbs but those waves are subtle and do not come into sight only through some medium they are reeled out of their subtlety.

"Likewise in human beings these qualities are hidden and only become manifest through an inward or outward medium—one person through speech, another through discord, another through war and peace. They cannot see human attributes: if they examine themselves, they will not find anything. So they suppose themselves empty of these attributes. Yet it is not the case that they have changed from what they were, only these things are hidden in us like the water in the sea. The waters leaves not the sea save through the medium of a cloud; they do not become visible except in a wave. The wave is a commotion visible from within us, without an external medium. But so long as the sea is still, they see nothing. Their body is on the shore of the sea and their soul is of the sea. Look at how many fishes and snakes and birds and creatures of all kinds come forth and show themselves and then return to the sea? Their attributes, such as anger and envy and lust and the rest, come forth from this sea. So they may say that their attributes are subtle lovers of God. They cannot perceive them save through the medium of the tongue; when they become naked, they do not see them because of their subtlety."

As they manifest gathering, they recognize, "There is no monkhood in Islam: the congregation is a mercy." The Messenger labored for solidarity since the gathering of spirits has a great and momentous effect whereas in singleness and isolation this is not achieved. That is the secret of why mosques were erected so that the inhabitants of the community might gather there and greater mercy and profit ensue. Houses are separate for the purpose of dispersion and the concealment of private relations—that is their use. Great mosques were erected so that the whole city might be assembled there. The Kabah was instituted in order that the greater part of mankind might gather there out of all cities and regions of the world.

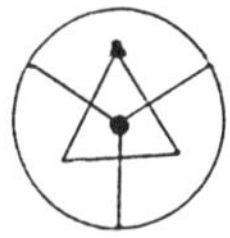

Wisdom

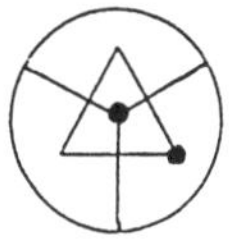

Courage

Through becoming the servant of God, spiritual warriors are thankful to God and humble before God's Will for only God is the Rich (al-Ghanī), the Enricher (al-Mughnī). They are in need of God alone so that in their relationships, they manifest wisdom and courage. In this way they are able to serve others not for the benefits that they may give them.

Their spiritual quest for true self arises out of a quest for that which has been found. There are two basic kinds of quests and the human quest usually consists in seeking a thing which they have not yet found. Night and day they are engaged in searching for that, whereas the quest where the thing has been found and the object attained is a strange quest indeed, surpassing human imagination, inconceivable to them. While the human quest is for something new which has not yet been found is for something they have found already and then seek. This is God's quest for God has found all things and all things are found in His power. He only has to say, "'*Be!' and it is*." He is the Finder, the Bountiful for God has found all things. Yet for all that God is the Seeker. "*He is the Seeker, the Prevailer*." The meaning of this is therefore, "Oh human being so long as you are engaged in the quest that is created in time, which is a human attribute, you remain far from that goal. When your quest passes away in God's quest and God's quest overrides your quest, then you become a seeker by virtue of God's quest."

This also allows spiritual warriors to open their heart in order to receive a Divine disposition to do good or to be benevolent. A disposition to do good creates a benevolent heart which becomes the mirror in which God's favors are manifest. When the Divine favors are manifest and come through them, when they feel His presence, they will feel shame at their improper actions. This causes both they and others to have a conscience. Thus their benevolence will protect them and others from wrongdoing. When the archangel Gabriel asked the Messenger, "What is divine benevolence?" The Messenger said, "To pray and glorify God as if you are in His presence, as if you see Him." Then the Messenger continued, "For if you are unable to see Him, He certainly sees you."

When they reach this level of realization of Divine benevolence, they will have consciously given birth to their conscience. They will feel that gaze of God upon them and will be ashamed to commit wrong.

The Messenger said, "Conscience is total good." If they as believers have conscience, they are aware of what they are doing and they cannot do wrong; when a heart is filled with conscience, the possessor of that heart encounters no harm either in this world or in the Hereafter. The Sign of their being with conscience is their lack of arrogance and self-importance. They never oppress or try to dominate others. Manifesting the sign of the Enricher (al-Mughnī) brings them material and spiritual richness so that they can satisfy the needs of the needy. It is related to the Merciful (al-Raḥmān), the Able (al-Qādir), and the Just (al-'Adl).

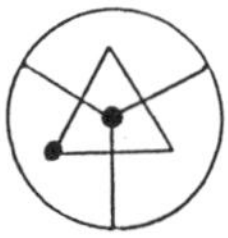

Temperance

Spiritual warriors learn to avoid and avert harm to the extent that those who are near to us are also protected from harmful things (*māni'*) as they manifest temperance. The quality is related to the Preserver (al-Ḥafiẓ). The

Quran says they may dislike what is good (5:216) or not be given what they ask for because God in His wisdom knows best and this is a manifestation of the sign al-Māni'.

Once a woman came to Caliph 'Alī crying, "One of my little ones has climbed up the water spout. If I call him, he won't come to my hand and if I leave him, I'm afraid he will fall to the ground. He isn't old enough to understand if I try to warn him. Please come and help me. Be quick, apply the cure for my heart is trembling.

"'Alī said, "Take another child up to the roof. When your little one will see someone his own age, he will come quickly from the water-spout to the other child."

The woman acted accordingly. When the infant saw the other child, he turned his face delightedly towards him and came to the roof from the back of the water-spout.

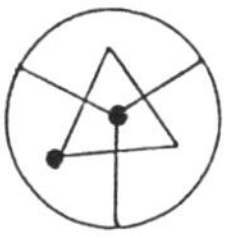

Temperance

At the same time, spiritual warriors may suffer through very difficult times and great pain as a means of educating themselves in their relations with others. Through the pain, the punisher (*ḍārr*), they learn patience, perseverance, courage, and steadfastness. Trying to actualize the quality of God's gifts to them, namely, intellect, conscience, and faith as tools whereby they are able to discern and discriminate between things, and chose His way. They awaken to, become aware and conscious of God's blessings (al-Nāfi', Creator of the Beneficial) as they manifest temperance. Seeing God's Will in the universe, spiritual warriors open their eyes to receive the good God has willed in the universe through their instinctive nature of attraction to pleasure.

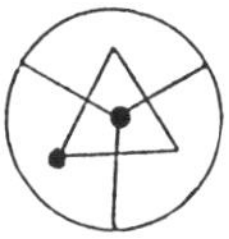

Temperance

Once there was a water carrier who owned a donkey. The donkey was bent double because of having carried such heavy loads. It yearned passionately for the day it should die. Barley? It never got its fill even of dry straw. Once day the royal stable master, who chanced to be acquainted with the donkey's owner, saw the donkey and took pity on it. He greeted the owner and asked how the donkey had been so broken.

"It's because of my poverty and lack of means," the man replied. "The dumb beast can't even get straw."

"Hand him over to me for a few days," said his friend. "He'll soon get strong in the royal stables."

So the man handed over his donkey and his compassionate friend took it to the Sultan's stables. There the donkey saw on every side Arab horses, well-fed and plump, fine and shinning as new pins. Under their feet the ground was swept and sprinkled with water. Straw was brought regularly and barley served at the proper time. It saw how the horses were curried and rubbed down.

"Most glorious Lord," the donkey cried, lifting up its muzzle, "am I not also your creature? I concede that I am but a donkey yet why am I so wretched, so thin, with sores on my back? At night what with the pain in my back and the hunger in my belly, I long every moment to die. These horses are so happy and well provided for. Why am I singled out for torture and trial?"

Suddenly came the rumor of war. It was time for the Arabs to be saddled and go into action. They were wounded by the arrows of the enemy. The shafts pierced them on every side. When the Arabs returned from the campaign they all collapsed and lay on their backs in the stable. Their legs were tightly bandaged with canvas strips; the attendants standing in file were probing their bodies with scalpels to extract the shafts from the wounds.

"God," cried the donkey, beholding this, "I am well content with being poor and preserved. I have no stomach for that fine fare and frightful wounds." The donkey clearly lacked a sense of temperance gained through abandoning things of this world.

CHAPTER TEN
SERVING AS A GUIDE AND TEACHER TO OTHERS

On their final stage towards growing closer to God, spiritual warriors manifest an inner light (*nūr*) when they recognize that their very being including the effects of their being like their knowledge, feelings, and behavior all come from God's light. The servant of God can become a guide (*hādī*) to the Straight Path, with a special quality that marks this person and makes them different from all others (*badi'*). They put aside all desires of this world as they engage in work that will be everlasting (*bāqī*). They recognize that everything they have is only temporarily theirs (*wārith*) and eventually will return to God. As right in guidance (*rashīd*), they become teachers of others; they are patient (*ṣabur*).

APPLICATION

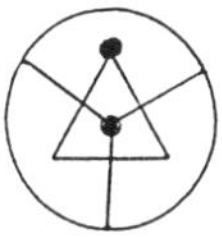

Wisdom

To manifest light (*nūr*) is to manifest wisdom and consciousness and to become as the Messenger prayed, "Oh My Lord, render me light." The servants know that all existence including their knowledge, feelings, and behavior come from God's light. In the verse of light, according to Algazel, five aspects of the self are symbolized:[1] the sensory, the imaginative, the intellectual, the rational, and the intuitive. The verse reads, "*God is the Light of the heavens and the earth; the likeness of His Light is as a niche* (sensory aspects of self), *wherein is a lamp. The lamp in a glass* (imaginative function), *the glass, as it were a glittering star* (the intellect), *kindled from a Blessed Tree* (reason), *an olive that is neither of the East nor of the West, whose oil wellnigh would shine even if no fire touched it* (intuition); *Light upon Light*" (24:35).

"The niche for a lamp in a wall symbolizes the sensory self for its lights come through several apertures, the eyes, ears, nostrils, etc. As to the imaginative aspect of self, it has three characteristics: first, its images consist of aspects of the material world because its images have definite and limited size, shape, and dimension and are definitely related to the subject in respect of distance. Also, one of the properties of a material substance, which has physical properties, is to be opaque to the light of the pure intellect, which transcends these categories of direction, quantity, and distance. Secondly, if that substance is clarified, refined, disciplined, and controlled, it attains to a correspondence with and a similarity to the ideas of the intellect, and becomes transparent to light from them. Thirdly, imagination is at first very much needed in order that intelligent knowledge may be controlled by it so that the knowledge be not disturbed, unsettled, and dissipated and so get out of hand. The images supplied by the imagination hold together the knowledge supplied by the intellect.

"Now in the world of everyday experience, the sole object in which they will find these three peculiarities in relation to physical light is glass for glass also is originally an opaque substance but is clarified and refined until it becomes transparent to the light of a lamp which indeed it transmits unaltered. Again, glass keeps the lamp from going out by a breeze of wind. What, then, could more appropriately symbolize imagination than a glass?

"Intellect gives cognizance of the Divine Ideas. The point of the symbolism must be obvious, it is the light-giving of the lamp. As for reason, it is to begin from one proposition, then to branch out into two when two becomes four and so on until by this process of logical division they become very numerous. It leads, finally, to conclusions which in their turn become germs producing like conclusions, these latter being also susceptible of continuation, each with each. The symbol which their world yields for this is a tree. And when further they consider that the fruit of the discursive reason is material for this multiplying, establishing, and fixing of all knowledge, it will naturally not be typified by trees like quince, apple, pomegranate, nor, in brief, by any other tree whatever except the olive. For the quintessence of the fruit of the olive is its oil which is the material which feeds the lamps and has this peculiarity, as against all other oils, that it increases radiance. Again, if people give the adjective blessed to specially fruitful tree, surely the tree the fruitfulness whereof is absolutely infinite should be named *blessed*! Finally, if the ramifications of those pure intellectual propositions do not admit of relation to direction and to distance, then perhaps a typical tree will be said to be *neither from the East nor from the West.*

"Intuition is possessed by saints as well as Prophets when it is absolutely luminous and clear. The thought-spirit is divided into that which needs be instructed, advised, and supplied from without if the acquisition of knowledge is to be continuous while a portion of it is absolutely clear, as though it were self-luminous and had no external source of supply. Applying these considerations, they see how justly this clear, strong natural faculty is described by the words, *Whose oil were wellnigh would shine even if no fire touched it* for there be saints whose light shines so bright that it is *wellnigh,* independent of that which Prophets supply while there be Prophets whose light is *well-nigh,* independent of that which angels supply. Such is the symbolism and aptly does it typify the class.

"And inasmuch as the lights of the human self are graded rank on rank, then that of sense comes first, the foundation and preparation for the imagination (for the latter can only be conceived as superimposed after sense); those of the intellect and discursive reason come thereafter. All which explains why the glass is, as it were, the place for the lamp's immanence and the niche, for the glass. That is to say, the lamp is within the glass and the glass within the niche. Finally, existence, as a graded succession of lights, explains the words of the text *Light upon Light....*

"But this symbolism holds only for the hearts of true

believers or of Prophets and saints, but not for the hearts of unbelievers for the term *light* is expressive of right-guidance alone. But as for the person who is turned from the path of guidance, he is false; he is darkness; nay, he is worse than this for darkness is natural. It leads one neither one way nor the other but the minds of unbelievers and the whole of their perceptions are perverse and support each other mutually in the actual deluding of their owners. They are like *shadows upon a fathomless sea covered by a wave above which is a wave above which are clouds, shadows piled one upon another...* (24:40)

"Now that fathomless sea is the world, this world of mortal dangers, of evil chances, of blinding trouble. The first *wave* is the wave of desires, whereby the self acquires the attraction to pleasure and is occupied with sensual pleasures and the satisfaction of worldly ambitions so that *they eat and luxuriate like cattle. Hell shall be their place of entertainment*!

"Well does this *wave* represent darkness therefore since love for the creature makes the self both blind and deaf. The second *wave* is the wave of the avoidance of pain which impels the soul to anger, wrath, enmity, hatred, prejudice, envy, boastfulness, ostentation, pride. Well is this, too, the symbol of darkness for wrath is the ego of a human being's intellect and well also is it the uppermost wave for anger is stronger even than desires, swelling anger diverts the self from even desires and makes it oblivious to enjoyment. Desires cannot for a moment stand up against anger at its height.

"Finally, *the cloud* is rank beliefs and lying heresies and corrupt imaginings which become so many veils veiling the unbeliever from the true faith, from knowledge of the Real, and from illumination by the sunlight of the Quran and human intelligence. For it is the property of a cloud to veil the shining of the sunlight. Now these things, being all of them darkness, are well called *darkness on darkness piled,* shutting the self out from the knowledge of things near, let alone things far away, veiling the unbeliever, therefore, from the apprehension of the miracles of the Prophet, though he is so near to grasp, so manifest upon the least reflection. truly it might be said of such a one that *'when he puts forth his hand, he can wellnigh see it not.'* Finally, if all these lights have, as they saw, their source and origin in the great primary, the one Real, then every believer in unity may well believe that *to whomsoever God assigns no light, no light has he* (24:40)."

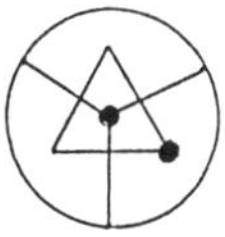

Courage

The response to "*Guide us on the Straight Path*" (1:5) is to become a guide (*hādī*) for others. In this way spiritual warriors become an instrument for others' salvation for they are charged with enforcing the Truth: What God commands and what God forbids. The degree of spiritual state which one may discover is due to the Messenger and his influence. In the first place, all gifts are showered on him then they are distributed from him to other people. Such is the rule. God said, "Oh Prophet, peace be upon you and God's mercy and blessings! They have scattered all gifts upon you." The Messenger said, "And upon God's righteous servants!"

God's way is exceeding fearful, blocked and—as it were—full of obstacles. The Messenger was the first to risk his life, leading his horse and pioneering the road. Whoever goes on this road does so by his guidance and guarding. He discovered the road in the first place and set up way marks everywhere, placing pieces of wood as if to say, "Do not go in this direction and do not go in that direction. If you go in that direction you will perish even as the people of 'Ad and Thamud and if you go in this direction you will be saved like the believers." All of the Quran expounds this for "*therein are clear Signs,*" that is to say, upon these ways they have given way marks. If they attempt to break any of these pieces of wood, all attack us, saying, "Why do you destroy the road for us and why do you labor to accomplish their destruction? Perchance you are a highwayman."

Spiritual warriors know that Muhammad is the guide. Unless spiritual warriors first comes to Muhammad, according to tradition, they cannot reach unto God. Similarly when they wish to go to a certain place, first reason leads the way, saying, "You must go to a certain place. That is in your best interests." After that the eyes act as a guide and then the limbs begin to move, all in that order, even though the limbs have no knowledge of the eye, neither the eye of reason.

A person of courage at the stage of the Guide in search of right guidance once shut himself up for a forty day retreat, seeking after a particular object. A voice came to him, saying, "Such a lofty object will never be attained by a forty day retreat. Abandon your discipline so that the look of a great saint may fall upon you and your object will be realized."

"Where shall I find that great one?" the man asked.

"In the congregational mosque," came the answer.

"How shall I recognize the person in such a crowd of people?"

"Go," he was told, "and he will recognize you and will look upon you. The sign that has looked upon you will be that the pitcher of water you are carrying will drop from your hand and you will become unconscious. Then you will know that he has looked upon you."

He acted accordingly. He filled a pitcher with water and went round the congregation in the mosque like a water-carrier. He was wandering between the ranks of the worshippers when suddenly he was seized with ecstasy. He uttered a loud cry and the pitcher fell from his hand. He remained in a corner of the mosque unconscious. All the people departed. When he came to his senses he saw that he was alone. He did not see the guide who had looked upon him, but he had gained his object.

There are certain men of God who because of their great majesty and jealousy for God do not show themselves openly; but they cause disciples to attain important objects and bestow gifts on them. Such mighty guides are rare and precious.

When they are marked by a special positive characteris-

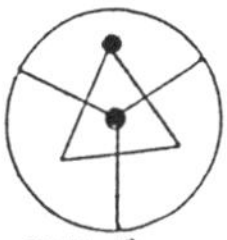

Wisdom

tics, they have manifest their portion of the Originator (al-Badī'). It is an ability to know, discover, and build things that others are not able to do.

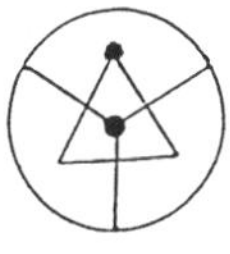

Wisdom

Through the manifestation of their portion of the Everlasting (al-Bāqī) and the success in detachment to material things of this world, they work for God's sake alone. They will then find that their work has an everlasting quality including something that will remain, confirm God's way, last, endure, and be relatively permanent for the worship of the servant is servitude to God.

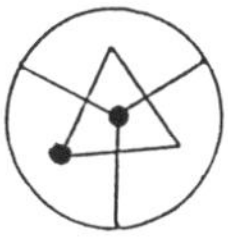

Temperance

Almost at the final level of the last stage of nearness to God, the servants perceive the truth of Divine Unity in the processes of creation and know that everything belongs to God and that God is the Inheritor (al-Warith) while they are only temporary custodians of His blessings including knowledge, wisdom, and guidance.

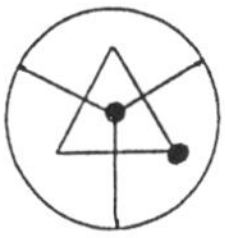

Courage

The last two levels are to manifest the signs the Right in Guidance (al-Rashīd) and the Patient (al-Ṣabur). As teachers of others, spiritual warriors teach but do not compel others to follow as they realize that everyone has a free will to accept or reject. They direct them to the right reason for why they should accept in order to bring their positive characteristics within into being. This would include their intentions, religious duties, and worldly affairs. Their teaching can become so effective when they manifest their portion of the Right in Guidance (al-Rashīd) that those that they teach will naturally follow God's Will because of their sense of justice and affection. The stages to the manifestation of this sign are: first of all, becoming conscious of what is being taught through the recognition that there is an underlying order both internal and external to them. Second, to help others to use their minds to discipline and educate their real self having died to their false self. Third, they learn God's Divine Law and live by it.

Spiritual warriors need to teach God's Word and good behavior to their children. They should secure for them conditions in which they can exercise what they have taught them. They do this without expecting any return from them. From the very beginning, they teach them to bear difficulty, to have patience, to think. They do not place in their hearts the love of the world. They teach them to dislike the things of this world that will render them proud—luxuries, beautiful clothes, delicacies, excess of ambition—because all of these, if obtained, will be subtracted from the good due them in the Hereafter. They try not to let them not get accustomed to good things. They try to break their bad habits and are aware that this, which may seem austere, should not bring forth in them the ugly character of miserliness towards their children. They should do it in respect and attachment to their faith.

The best teachers are those whose students see their teacher's will, power, generosity, love, and compassion and love them because of it, live to do what the teacher says, love to work for their satisfaction. Once of the best teachers traditionally has been Solomon who it is said was taught the language of the birds. Rūmī describes this ability of a teacher to respond in a particular way to each student.

Approach, oh Solomon,
    you that know the language of the birds
Sound the note of every bird that draws near.
When God sent you to the birds,
He taught you first the notes of all the birds.
To the predestinarian bird talk predestination,
To the bird with broken wings, preach patience,
To the patient well-doer preach comfort and
    pardon,
To the spiritual, mythical bird ('Anqā) relate the
    glories of the sacred mountain (Qāf),
To the pigeon preach avoidance of the hawk,
To the lordly hawk mercy and self-control;
As for the bat, who lingers helpless in the dark,
Acquaint him with the society of the light.
To the fighting partridge teach peace,
To the cock the signs of dawning day.
In this way deal with all from the hoopoe to the
    eagle.

Finally the Patient (al-Ṣabur). The Traditions say that Abu Mūsā narrated that the Messenger said, "None is more patient than God against harmful sayings. God hears from the people that they ascribe children to God yet God gives them health and supplies them with provisions."[2]

In another Tradition, 'Abdullāh narrated that the Messenger divided and distributed something as he used to do for some of the spoils of war that he received. One of the helpers (*anṣār*) said, "There should be no part for God in this distribution." I said, "I will mention this to the Messenger." So I went to him while he was sitting with hid Companions and quietly told him what the helper had said. The color of his face changed and he became so angry that I wished I had not told him. Then he said, "Moses was harmed more than this yet he remained patient."[3]

Here patience has developed out of courage, that is, developing the ability to withstand hardship, adversity, and stress. The servants attain patience through the rational function of counseling others to the positive to affirm their faith or rational resolve and to control the use of their inappropriate anger or desires. When they are caught in the dilemma between two opposing motives of self—one trying to counsel the self to patience and the other waiting impulsive behavior—they have to learn to chose a delayed response. This is patience—doing everything in its proper time and just the way it should be done. Patience is a high state for a believer. Neither success nor perfection can be achieved without pain. Pain of the flesh is hasty in what it wants, is lazy in working for what it wants, does not know the right measure of things, and wants more than it needs. The servants who are in equilibrium and moderation neither delay nor hasten but act in a determined time. They are patient in their continuous battle with their ego and they persevere in God's commands.

Once a child who lived in the desert said to his mother, "On dark nights a horrible demon appears to me and I am terribly afraid."

"Don't be afraid," said his mother. "The next time you see that form, attack it bravely. Then it will become clear that it is nothing but a fantasy."

"But mother," said the child, "what if the demon's mother has given him similar advice? What shall I do if she has counseled him, saying, 'Don't say a word so that you won't be exposed?' How shall I recognize him then?"

"Keep silent and yield to him and wait with patience," his mother answered. "It may be that some word may leap from his mouth. Or if it does not leap, it may be that from your tongue some word may leap involuntarily or in your thoughts some words or some idea may spring up so that out of that idea or those words you will know him for what he is. For then you will have been affected by him. That is the reflection of him and his feelings that has sprung up inside of you."

One day a healer was speaking about patience when a scorpion stung him several times. Finally he was asked, "Why didn't you drive it away?" He replied, "I was too ashamed to do anything because I was speaking of patience."

CONCLUSION

Through the journey of the spiritual warrior of knowledge-process-actions of assuming a portion of the Most Beautiful Names, the interactional quality of God's Will operative in nature's method of operation becomes clear. In the Islamic understanding of God's workings in the universe, creation is not conceived as having been a one time "big bang," from which God then withdrew. Rather, creation in the Islamic perspective is seen as an ongoing process whereby all life pulsates with each breath, dying and being reborn with every expansion and contraction.

While this work analyzed each of the Ninety-Nine Most Beautiful Names as they have been encountered by spiritual warriors throughout history, depending on whether they were at the stage of knowledge (theoethics), process (psychoethics) or action (socioethics), it seems only fair to finally understand the synthetic, interactional quality of God's Will in nature where the richness of the multiplicity of possibilities never loses the sense of oneness, unity and balance.

In Part II: The Process of Moral Healing for Spiritual Warriors Through Psychoethics, the spiritual warrior takes the knowledge of Part I: Nourishment of Spiritual Warriors: Knowledge of God Through Theoethics, as spiritual nourishment to be "consumed" in order to transform the self and assume a portion of the Ninety-Nine Most Beautiful Names. Three aspects of self are separately disciplined.

Attraction to pleasure which is the instinctive, animal urge to preserve the species, is disciplined through acquiring temperance. Temperance comes from assuming a portion of the Most Beautiful Names which God Self-disclosed to creation. This results in spiritual warriors out of free choice and love for God, giving to others what they themselves need (*ithār*). This occurs through seven stages: Resolve, Hope-Fear, Piety, Moderation, Tranquillity,

Spiritual Poverty and Self-Restraint.

Avoidance of harm/pain is the instinctive, animal urge to preserve the individual. It is disciplined through acquiring courage and/or trust in God. Courage comes from assuming a portion of the Most Beautiful Names which God Self-disclosed to humanity. There are seven stages: Compassion, Moral Reasonableness, Thankfulness, Vigilance, Trust, Repentance and Patience.

Reason is the instinctive, angelic urge to preserve the eternal possibility of self. This can only happen if reason disciplines the two animal instincts of attraction to pleasure and avoidance of harm/pain. Out of this wisdom develops which for the spiritual warrior is belief in the One God. This is enhanced by assuming a portion of the Names and Qualities through which God Self-disclosed to Self and develops through seven stages: Aspiration, Self-Examination, Truthfulness, Contentment, Unity, Sincerity and Remembrance.

The final proof of the effects of the process come through socioethics—how spiritual warriors relate to other people with a sense of fairness and justice which others acknowledge in the spiritual warrior. Proof of the success or failure of the stage of process (psychoethics) is seen in socioethics. This has ten stages:

In the first stage of Part III: The Actions of Spiritual Warriors: Proof of Moral Healing Through Socioethics, spiritual warriors learn about socially awakening to the noble character traits manifest through God's Most Beautiful Names. This awakening strengthens them in being able to empty their heart of everything but the desire to draw closer to God in order to enhance their relationships with others. When their heart is emptied of ego and negative traits, their mercy precedes their wrath towards all of creation (*raḥmān*) and they are compassionate (*raḥīm*) towards believers. With their heart empty of ego, their instinctive functions of inappropriate anger and desires are able to be controlled by reason in their relationships with others, manifesting the sign of being a sovereign (*malik*) over the self. Reason becomes the dominate force in their relations with them. The emptied heart is then cleansed (*quddūs*) of pre-judgments, stereotyping of others or prejudice and discrimination towards others. Their heart fills with a healthy view of others (*salām*), having eliminated their negative attitudes towards them. During this initial stage of the awakening and effacing of ego, spiritual warriors seek refuge in God the Giver of Faith (ya-Mu'min) for the fear, stress, and pain that accompanies the loss of their false identity or ego. They seek refuge from their failures as they may still try to possess and control others instead of reasoning with them. They are then able to relate to others without fear because God, the Giver of Faith (al-Mu'min), is their refuge. Guarding against wronging others (*muhaymin*), seeking to overcome the powers which may try to divide them from their friends (*'azīz*), implementing God's Will (*jabbār*), and effacing any egotism or pride (*mutakabbir)* that may remain with them are the final signs to manifest in their relations with others in their socially awakening to trying to assume noble character traits.

Spiritual warriors enter the creative process in stage two of socioethics in their attempt to grow closer to God. Being creative is to be able to conceive of the possibilities inherent within things that God gave through their natural disposition (*fiṭrat Allāh*). Manifesting their portion of the Sign, the Creator (ya-Khāliq), they move towards fostering their relationships with others. How they shape these friendships into a unique beauty (ya-Muṣawwir) will show the extent to which they manifest the Maker of Perfect Harmony (ya-Bāri'). They begin the recreation of the self or return to their true self being a forgiver (*ghaffār*) of those who have wronged them. If they manifest this Sign, they will no longer point out imperfections or faults of believers. They will try to cover over their imperfections rather than indicate them. They pray for their own wrongdoings and a Sign of their having been forgiven will be when they no longer commit the mistakes they had previously made.

In their return to the true self, the rational function of spiritual warriors should be in control over their emotions and behavior, their attraction to pleasure and avoidance of harm. It is then that they will manifest their portion of ya-Qahhār.

Others to whom spiritual warriors relate are then safe from their irrationality. With this in mind, as they begin to control their self through their cognitive or rational function, they begin to be a bestower (*wahhāb*) of what they have to those in need without thought of compensation. Seeking spiritual sustenance and nourishment (ya-Razzāq) to sustain them through the return, spiritual warriors appeal to God the Opener (ya-Fattāḥ) to open their hearts to His mercy and generosity; to the Knower (ya-'Alīm) for knowledge that can only come from God. This knowledge is called *irfān* (gnosis, mysticism).

A sign of the creative unfolding of their portion of the Provider (ya-Razzāq) is when spiritual warriors find others are dependent upon them because they use their words to direct them to the Straight Path and to teach them God's Word without personally gaining any material benefit from them. When they attain a sense of flexibility in facing their problems and solving them in a creative way, they will know they are manifesting their portion of the Sign the Opener (ya-Fattāḥ). When they come to experience intuitive knowledge and come to know the Truth as the Truth, they will have been able to fully enter the creative process by manifesting their portion of the Sign the Knower (ya-'Alīm). They are ready for stage three, counseling the self to the positive and trying to prevent the development of the negative.

In the third stage of the manifestation of the signs within and without spiritual warriors learned to counsel themselves and others to the positive, trying to prevent the development of the negative. Although apparently opposites—attraction/ repulsion or avoidance—as they move through the third stage they recognize an underlying healthy tension between them. They become a constrictor (*qābiḍ*) one moment and the next, an expander (*bāsiṭ*). They turn from falsity (*khāfiḍ*) to praising truthfulness (*rāfi'*), raising their friends to positions of honor (*mu'izz*) while they humble themselves *(mudhill)*, guide others towards perfection (sami') as they behold the signs in creation *(baṣiṭ)*. Strengthened by these tensions, they can now counsel themselves to truth and justice (*ḥakam)*, place things in positions appropriate to them (*'adl*), relate to others with gentleness (*laṭīf*) and compassion as they are rewarded with consciousness (*khābir*).

Manifesting the moral reasonableness of a religiously cultured person, spiritual warriors recognize their goal of perfection of the self. Without morality, there can be no perfection. Without self-discipline there can be no morality. They recognize they need to be a forebearer (*ḥalīm*), not quick to judgment and judging others. Their moral reasonableness causes them to reflect on what they consider to be magnificent (*'aẓiz*) about themselves which may lead them to self-conceit, vanity and arrogance towards others. Instead they need to die to the false self, their false sense of their own magnificence, in order to be freed from the cage of the body and perfect their real self. They strengthen their faith as religiously cultured monotheists in order to enhance the possibility of response to their being a concealer of faults (*ghafur*) of others and being thankful (*shakūr*) to God for their blessings. They continue their innate sense of generosity towards others making sure, as part of their covenant with God, that it is done for the sake of God alone (*'alī)*, for His satisfaction. They consciously strive to follow the *sunnah*. Their goal is to exhibit model behavior towards others. They seek God's protection as they try to be a protector (*ḥafiẓ*) of those around them, recognizing that at any moment He could choose to take them back to Him. Whatever spiritual warriors have is but temporary in preparation for the eternal. They seek to be a maintainer (*muqiṭ*) of God's Will in their relations with others and not the will of this or that person. Finally, they act as a reckoner (*ḥasīb*) doing a daily accounting of their deeds before the day of the final accounting as the final level of stage four in their journey towards assuming the noble character traits.

Spiritual power comes from being majestic (*jalīl*). This power manifests itself in various signs within them. Each sign empowers more majesty to them: being generous (*karīm*) and vigilant (*raqīb*), responding to the requests of others (*mujīb*) in need, gaining extensive (*wāsi'*) knowledge of the world and self, becoming wise (*ḥakīm*), giving through their sense of loving (*wadūd*) to others what they need themselves, perfecting of their moral qualities (*majīd*), giving life through knowledge, bearing witness to the visible and invisible alike (*shahīd*), and the power to sense the Real, the Truth (ya-Ḥaqq).

As God's trustee (*wakīl*) of nature and the universe, spiritual warriors become strong (*qawī*) and firm (*matīn*) in defeating their enemies within and carrying out their trusteeship without, becoming a friend (*walī*) to God's friends. They now have the strength to avoid the negative and be attracted to the praiseworthy (*ḥamīd*) as they are a reckoner (*muḥṣī*) for their wrongdoings, seeking an understanding of the Originator (ya-Mubdi') and the Restorer (ya-Mu'id). Cleansing their hearts of worldly desires (*muḥyī*). As they move towards perfection of their character/perception, spiritual warriors become the slayer (*mumīt*) of their false self while becoming conscious of their true, living (*ḥayy*) self. Gaining a sense of objectivity (*qayyūm*) in their relations to others by detaching their hearts from everything other than God, spiritual warriors express a richness of character (*majīd*). Perfecting their perception and character as they move towards unifying (*wāḥid, aḥad*) their inner and outer self, they become a model (*ṣamad*) for others.

Spiritual warriors realize they are able (*qadīr /muqtadir*) to perfect their actions and direct their motivations towards assuming the noble character traits in their relations with others when they empower themselves. They pray to the Promoter (ya-Muqaddim) to advance them and those to whom they relate on the path and not to fall under the power of the Postponer (ya-Mu'akhkhir) because of their actions or weakness of motivation. They take the initiative, becoming first *(awwal)* in their devotions and last (*ākhir*) in reproaching others for their faults, without first recognizing their own. They then manifest (*ẓāhir*) their inner, hidden (*bāṭin*) qualities that have been transformed through this process, seeking the help of the Governor (ya-Wālī) to control their 'self' from rebelling against God's commands. They confess their belief (*muta'ālī*) in God by doing good (*barr*) to others in need, being a repenter (*tawwāb*) of their past mistakes and being an avenger (*muntaqim*) towards the enemy within. Spiritual warriors erase ('*afu*) the wrongdoings done to them by others in the final stage of perfecting their actions and motivations.

At the stage of servanthood, having relinquished what they considered to be their 'will' and becoming one with God's Will, which is to seek to know their 'self' and thereby become conscious of God, spiritual warriors manifest being clement (*ra'ūf*) towards others, bearing witness to God's power (*mālik al-mulk*). They find certainty of faith in God's majesty and bounty (*dhū 'l-jalāl wa 'l-ikrām*). As God's servant, they demand justice (*muqsiṭ*) for others, unite (*jāmi'*) the similar and dissimilar in their relations with others, serving others as spiritually rich (*ghanī/mughnī*), avoiding the negative and harmful (*māni'*) while they realize that they grow through experiencing pain and hardship (*ḍārr*) as well as the beneficial and pleasure (*nāfi'*) as God's Will operates in the universe.

At the last stage, spiritual warriors manifest an inner light (*nūr*) as they recognize that all their knowledge, feelings, and behavior come from God's Light. They move closer to being a guide (*hadī*) for others because they now manifest a quality that distinguishes them from others (*bādī*‘), engaging themselves in work that is considered to be everlasting (*bāqī*) because everything they have returns to the Inheritor (ya-Warith). As the right in guidance (*rashīd*) and guide to right behavior, they are patient (*ṣabur*).

A: List of The Order of the 99 Most Beautiful Names, Translation, Transliteration, Quality and Number Symbolism (West and East)

Order	Translation	Transliteration	Quality	ABJAD W	E
1	Merciful, The	al-Raḥmān	B	298	298
2	Compassionate, The	al-Raḥīm	B	258	258
3	Sovereign, The	al-Malik	C	90	90
4	Holy, The	al-Quddūs	C	410	170
5	Flawless, The	al-Salām	H	371	131
6	Faith, The Giver of	al-Mu'min	H	136	136
7	Guardian, The	al-Muhaymin	H	145	145
8	Incomparable, The	al-'Azīz	C	94	94
9	Compeller, The	al-Jabbār	B	206	206
10	Proud, The	al-Mutakabbir	H	662	662
11	Creator, The	al-Khāliq	C	731	731
12	Maker of Perfect Harmony, The	al-Bāri'	H	213	213
13	Shaper of Unique Beauty, The	al-Muṣawwir	H	306	336
14	Forgiver, The	al-Ghaffār	B	1181	1181
15	Subduer, The	al-Qahhār	B	306	306
16	Bestower, The	al-Wahhāb	H	14	14
17	Provider, The	al-Razzāq	C	308	308
18	Opener, The	al-Fattāḥ	H	489	489
19	Knower, The	al-'Alīm	B	150	150
20	Constrictor, The	al-Qabid	H	193	903
21	Expander, The	al-Bāsiṭ	B	312	72
22	Abaser, The	al-Khāfiḍ	H	771	1481
23	Exalter, The	al-Rāfi'	B	351	351
24	Honorer, The	al-Mu'izz	C	117	117
25	Dishonorer, The	al-Mudhill	H	770	770
26	All-Hearing, The	al-Samī'	H	420	180
27	All-Seeing, The	al-Baṣīr	H	272	302
28	Arbiter, The	al-Ḥakam	C	68	68
29	Just, The	al-'Adl	C	104	104
30	Subtle, The	al-Laṭīf	H	129	129
31	Aware, The	al-Khabīr	B	812	812
32	Forebearing, The	al-Ḥalīm	B	88	88
33	Magnificent, The	al-'Aẓīm	B	920	1020
34	Concealer of Faults, The	al-Ghafūr	B	1186	1186
35	Thankfulness, The Rewarder of	al-Shakūr	B	1226	526
36	Highest, The	al-'Alī	C	110	110

Key to Quality: B = Balanced, C = Cold, H = Hot

A: List of The Order of the 99 Most Beautiful Names, Translation, Transliteration, Quality and Number Symbolism (West and East)

Order	Translation	Transliteration	Quality	ABJAD	W/E
37	Great, The	al-Kabīr	B	232	232
38	Preserver, The	al-Ḥafīẓ	B	898	998
39	Maintainer, The	al-Muqīt	H	550	550
40	Reckoner, The	al-Ḥasīb	B	320	80
41	Majestic, The	al-Jalīl	C	73	73
42	Generous, The	al-Karīm	B	270	270
43	Vigilant, The	al-Raqīb	B	312	312
44	Prayer, The Responder to	al-Mujīb	H	55	55
45	Vast, The	al-Wāsī	B	377	137
46	Wise, The	al-Ḥakīm	B	78	78
47	Loving, The	al-Wadūd	B	20	20
48	Glorious, The	al-Majīd	B	57	57
49	Resurrector, The	al-Bā'ith	B	573	573
50	Witness, The	al-Shahīd	H	1019	319
51	Truth, The	al-Ḥaqq	C	108	108
52	Trustee, The	al-Wakīl	B	66	66
53	Strong, The	al-Qawī	H	116	116
54	Firm, The	al-Matīn	H	500	500
55	Friend, The	al-Walī	H	46	46
56	Praised, The	al-Ḥamīd	B	62	62
57	Appraiser, The	al-Muḥṣī	H	118	148
58	Beginner, The	al-Mubdi'	H	56	56
59	Restorer, The	al-Mu'īd	B	124	124
60	Life-Giver, The	al-Muḥyī	H	68	68
61	Slayer, The	al-Mumīt	H	490	490
62	Living, The	al-Ḥayy	B	18	18
63	Self-Existing, The	al-Qayyūm	H	156	156
64	Resourceful, The	al-Wājid	B	14	14
65	Noble, The	al-Mājid	B	48	48
66	Unique, The	al-Wāḥid	B	19	19
67	One, The	al-Aḥad	C	13	13
68	Eternal, The	al-Samad	H	104	134
69	Able, The	al-Qādir	C	305	305
70	Powerful, The	al-Muqtadir	C	744	744
71	Promoter, The	al-Muqaddim	C	184	184
72	Postponer, The	al-Mu'akhkhir	B	846	846
73	First, The	al-Awwal	H	37	37
74	Last, The	al-Ākhir	C	801	801
75	Manifest, The	al-Ẓahir	B	1006	1106

A: List of The Order of the 99 Most Beautiful Names, Translation, Transliteration, Quality and Number Symbolism (West and East)

Order	Translation	Transliteration	Quality	ABJAD W/E	
76	Hidden, The	al-Bāṭin	H	62	62
77	Governor, The	al-Wālī	H	47	47
78	Exalted, The	al-Muta'āliā	H	551	551
79	Goodness, The Source				
	of All	al-Barr	B		
80	Repentance, The			202	202
	Acceptor of	al-Tawwāb	H	409	409
81	Avenger, The	al-Muntaqim	H	630	630
82	Pardoner, The	al-'Afū	H	156	156
83	Clement, The	al-Ra'ūf	H	286	286
84	King of Absolute				
	Sovereignty	Mālik al-Mulk	B	212	212
85	Lord of Majesty and	Dhū 'l-Jalāl			
	Generosity	wa 'l-Ikrām	B	1100	1100
86	Equitable, The	al-Muqsiṭ	B	449	209
87	Gatherer, The	al-Jāmi'	B	114	114
88	Rich, The	al-Ghanī	H	960	1060
89	Enricher, The	al-Mughnī	H	1000	1100
90	Protector, The	al-Māni'	H	161	161
91	Punisher, The	al-Ḍārr	H	291	1001
92	Creator of the Beneficial,		H		
	The	al-Nāfi'	H	201	201
93	Light, The	al-Nūr	H	256	256
94	Guide, The	al-Hādī	H	20	20
95	Originator, The	al-Badī'	B	86	86
96	Everlasting, The	al-Bāqī	H	113	113
97	Inheritor, The	al-Wārith	B	707	707
98	Right in Guidance, The	al-Rashīd	B	1214	514
99	Patient, The	al-Ṣabur	H	268	298

B: List of the Translation of the 99 Most Beautiful Names with the Order, Division and Summary Description of Role in Theoethics, Psychoethics and Socioethics

Translation	Theoethics	Psychoethics	Socioethics
22 Abaser, The (Creation)	Abases unbelievers by means of misfortune; isolates them from Him.	Hope/Fear	Abase idol/ego in relations with others.
69 Able, The (Self)	Power comes from Will and Knowledge, causes things to happen; created everything by Himself without assistance of another.	Unity	Empowering the self and others to attain to unity in their relationships.
26 All-Hearing, The (Self)	Nothing escapes the All-Hearing including silence.	Self-Examination	Guarding against backbiting; listen to the Word of God.
27 All-Seeing, The (Self)	Watches and observes everything.	Self-Examination	Sense the Presence of the All-Seeing in relations with others.
57 Appraiser, The (Creation)	Analyzing, counting, recording qualities.	Piety	Reproach the self in relations with others.
28 Arbiter, The (Self)	No one overturns God's decisions or corrects them; arranges causes to effects; divine decree (cause) and predestination (effect).	Self-Examination	Foster truth and justice in relationships.
81 Avenger, The (Humanity)	Breaks the back of the arrogant; punishes criminals; intensifies punishment of tyrants.	Repentance	Take revenge against God's enemies.
31 Aware, The (Self)	No unconscious content hidden without the Aware knowing.	Self-Examination	Develops consciousness and awareness in relations with others.
58 Beginner, The (Creation)	Begins Creation.	Moderation	Understands beginnings.
16 Bestower, The (Humanity)	Gives freely without compensation or interest.	Moral Reasonablness	Give good to others who are in need and worthy without thought of compensation or self-interest.

B: List of the Translation of the 99 Most Beautiful Names with the Order, Division and Summary Description of Role in Theoethics, Psychoethics and Socioethics

Translation	Theoethics	Psychoethics	Socioethics
83 Clement, The (Humanity)	God has pity as an intensification of His Mercy.	Patience	Intense compassion for others.
2 Compassionate, The (Humanity)	Compassion towards the believers.	Compassion	Compassion towards the believers.
9 Compeller,The (Creation)	Effective in Will Power over everything; compels instinct to counsel to the positive and try to prevent the development of the negative.	Resolve	Enforce God's Will.
34 Concealer of Faults, The (Humanity)	Forgives and conceals faults from the hidden world.	Moral Reasonableness	Conceal the faults of others.
20 Constrictor, The (Creation)	Takes souls at the time of death; withholds sustenance.	Hope/Fear	Pray for patience.
92 Creator of the Beneficial, The (Creation)	Secondary cause created is being beneficial.	Self-Restraint	Being beneficial to others.
11 Creator, The (Creation)	Creates.	Resolve	Conceive of possibilities in things.
25 Dishonorer, The (Creation)	Dishonors at the Resurrection.	Hope/Fear	Dishonor God's enemies.
89 Enricher, The (Humanity)	Supplies everyone what they need.	Patience	Give to others in need what they need.
86 Equitable,The (Creation)	Acts and distributes justice to those who have been wronged.	Spiritual Poverty/ Altruism	Sense of measure seeing things in a fair way.
68 Eternal, The (Self)	Meets needs in accord with needs; satisfies as they should be met and not as one may want.	Unity	Become models for others by educating them.
96 Everlasting, The (Self)	Applies only to God Who is beyond time.	Remembrance	Bring an everlasting quality to our relationships when formed as a form of worship for God's sake alone.

B: List of the Translation of the 99 Most Beautiful Names with the Order, Division and Summary Description of Role in Theoethics, Psychoethics and Socioethics

Translation	Theoethics	Psychoethics	Socioethics
78 Exalted, The (Self)	Highest in intensified form; no defects of aging.	Remembrance	Understand the Signs within and without in relations with others.
23 Exalter, The (Creation)	Exalts believers by means of good fortune; draws them near to Him.	Hope/Fear	Treat friends of God as friends.
21 Expander, The (Creation)	Gives souls at the time of inception; makes substance plentiful—gifts, kindness, beauty.	Hope/Fear	Being thankful when in a state of expansion, joy.
6 Faith, The Giver of (Humanity)	Gives safety and security; blocks avenues of fear of any other than God.	Compassion	Seek refuge in Giver of Faith from the fear, stress and pain that accompanies the loss of our idol/ego.
54 Firm, The (Self)	Intensity of strength—cannot be saved from it or oppose it.	Contentment	Develop a receptiveness to empowerment in relations with others to work towards healing the self.
73 First, The (Self)	The first.	Sincerity	Be first in devotion so that others learn from that model.
5 Flawless, The (Self)	Lacks any imperfection.	Aspiration	Develop a healthy view of others having eliminated negative attitudes towards them.
32 Forebearer, The (Humanity)	Shows neither anger nor rage upon witnessing disobedience; no swift action taken.	Moral Reasonableness	Need self-discipline to proceed towards moral healing of self and others.
14 Forgiver, The (Humanity)	Manifests what is noble; hides what is disgraceful.	Compassion	Conceal faults of friends from others; forgive those who have wronged you.
55 Friend, The (Humanity)	Help others; God subdues His enemies and helps His friends.	Trust	Develop friendships with the friends of God.

B: List of the Translation of the 99 Most Beautiful Names with the Order, Division and Summary Description of Role in Theoethics, Psychoethics and Socioethics

Translation	Theoethics	Psychoethics	Socioethics
87 Gatherer, The (Creation)	Joins similar and dissimilar; opposites.	Spiritual Poverty/ Altruism	Gather behavior towards others and truths in one's heart.
42 Generous, The (Humanity)	Forgives although could punish; keeps promises and exceeds others in giving.	Thankfulness/ Generosity	Show generosity towards others.
48 Glorious, The (Self)	Noble in Essence; beautiful in Acts; generous in gifts.	Truthfulness	Seeking a noble essence; develop goodness of actions and generosity in giving to others in need.
79 Goodness, The Source of All (Self)	Punishes only for deeds done; rewards for good done are greater.	Remembrance	Be a doer of good among people.
77 Governor, The (Creation)	Plans the affairs of creation and assumes control over them.	Spiritual Poverty/ Altruism	Rule over others according to God's Commands.
37 Great, The (Self)	Perfection of Essence; perpetuity of past and future and all that exists comes from It; perfect and great.	Truthfulness	Human perfection lies in reason, piety, knowledge of God.
7 Guardian, The (Humanity)	Evolution and growth of creation through knowledge, control, protection.	Compassion	Guard against wronging others; keep control of situation; obtain rights for others; help friends stay on the Straight Path.
94 Guide, The (Humanity)	Guides to knowledge of the creation to things good for humanity.	Patience	Guide self and others to knowledge.
76 Hidden, The (Self)	The hidden.	Sincerity	Invite others to spiritual perfection.
36 Highest, The (Self)	No rank about It in terms of rank or space.	Truthfulness	To be detached and removed to a certain extent to allow for some objectivity in relationships; supporting and helping others for God's sake alone.

B: List of the Translation of the 99 Most Beautiful Names with the Order, Division and Summary Description of Role in Theoethics, Psychoethics and Socioethics

Translation	Theoethics	Psychoethics	Socioethics
4 Holy, The (Self)	Without blemish, shortcoming, weakness; above what perception can perceive.	Aspiration	Cleanse heart of prejudgments and stereotyping of others.
24 Honorer, The (Creation)	God gives dominion to those who recognize His Presence; grants contentment so human beings become needless; provides strength and support to control disposition; raises to honor in the Hereafter.	Hope/Fear	Raise friends to a position of honor.
8 Incomparable, The (Self)	Incomparable in importance, usefulness, inaccessibility.	Aspiration	Seek victory over powers that divide us from friends; control these powers in our relationship so it becomes incomparabale.
97 Inheritor, The (Creation)	Possessions return to the Inheritor after the passing away of the temporary owner.	Self-Restraint	Recognize that everything belongs to God.
29 Just, The (Self)	No fault in creation; dazzling symmetry and systematic order.	Self-Examination	Give rights in right measure; Signs within and without.
84 King of Absolute Sovereignty (Creation)	Carries out God's Will; brings into being, destroys, perpetuates, annihilates.	Spiritual Poverty/ Altruism	Govern as God's vicegerent.
19 Knower, The (Self)	Knows the hidden and manifest; small and great; before and after.	Self-Examination	Pray for intuitive knowledge not learned from any human source.
74 Last, The (Self)	The last.	Sincerity	Always remember the end and the return to God.
60 Life-Giver, The (Creation)	Brings life into being.	Moderation	Return to nature originated by God by ridding self of worldly desires.

B: List of the Translation of the 99 Most Beautiful Names with the Order, Division and Summary Description of Role in Theoethics, Psychoethics and Socioethics

Translation	Theoethics	Psychoethics	Socioethics
93 Light, The (Self)	Light-existence.	Remembrance	Render self and others light.
62 Living, The (Self)	Acts and perceives—no perceived thing strays from God's knowledge and no action from God's action.	Contentment	Our aliveness in our relations with others is determined by our perception and motivation to action.
85 Lord of Majesty and Generosity (Self)	All majesty and perfection belong to God; personality, glory,	Remembrance	Tied to each other through needs.
47 Loving, The (Humanity)	Desires good for all humanity; praises and rewards believers; does not require neediness on our part; mercy and grace transcend love; unconditional love.	Vigilance	Desire for others what desire for self.
33 Magnificent, The (Self)	That which human intellect cannot conceivably completely grasp the core of Its real nature; exceeds the limits of human understanding.	Truthfulness	Cultivate inner greatness, magnificence and strength in relations with others; die to false self.
39 Maintainer, The (Humanity)	Conveys nourishment through food to maintain the status quo; requires knowledge and power.	Thankfulness/ Generosity	Help maintain others in need.
41 Majestic, The (Self)	Includes strength, dominion, holiness, knowledge, wealth, power.	Truthfulness	Do not abuse your position of strength in relations with others.
12 Maker of Perfect Harmony, The (Creation)	In perfect harmony.	Resolve	Strive for perfect harmony in relations with others.
75 Manifest,The (Self)	Everything manifest comes from God.	Sincerity	Recognize the manifest in relations with others.

B: List of the Translation of the 99 Most Beautiful Names with the Order, Division and Summary Description of Role in Theoethics, Psychoethics and Socioethics

Translation	Theoethics	Psychoethics	Socioethics
1 Merciful, The (Humanity)	Universal mercy; mercy precedes wrath.	Compassion	Our mercy precede our wrath towards all of creation.
65 Noble, The (Self)	Nobility through kindness; glorifies, rewards, protects rights, solves difficulties.	Contentment	Find what God wants us to find in relations with others.
67 One, The (Self)	Indivisible reflects multiplicity in unity. Like geometric center, cannot be separated or duplicated.	Unity	Unity incomparable to anything inside or outside.
18 Opener, The (Humanity)	Opens things closed; clears things unclear; brings about victory; makes decisions known; discloses what is concealed.	Moral Reasonableness	Open knots, remove sadness and depression from the heart; remove doubts from the mind in relations with others.
95 Originator, The (Self)	Original—nothing similar, unequalled, incomparable.	Remembrance	Special positive characteristic—know, discover and build things not known before.
82 Pardoner, The (Humanity)	Erases wrongdoings and disregards disobedience.	Repentance	Seek pardon from God for wrongdoings done to you by others.
99 Patient, The (Humanity)	Does not act in haste or prematurely; acts in a determined measure and with a definite plan.	Patience	Not acting hastily or prematurely in relations with others.
72 Postponer, The (Creation)	Distances from Self those who are enemies.	Tranquillity	Be aware of temptations of the idol/ego.
70 Powerful, The (Creation)	Not only creates all power but has total control over it.	Tranquillity	Purify the self of greed and covetousness.
56 Praised, The (Self)	Majesty, exaltation, pefection in relation to those who praise God.	Contentment	Thoughts praise God.

B: List of the Translation of the 99 Most Beautiful Names with the Order, Division and Summary Description of Role in Theoethics, Psychoethics and Socioethics

Translation	Theoethics	Psychoethics	Socioethics
44 Prayer, The Responder to (Humanity)	Responds to those who ask even before an appeal is made.	Vigilance	Be sensitive to the needs of friends and respond to them before they ask.
38 Preserver, The (Creation)	Perpetuating the existence of existing things, sustaining them and safeguarding them from that which is inherently opposite and guarding and preserving the servants against wrongdoing.	Piety	Guarding and preserving the self and others from harm—physical and spiritual.
71 Promoter, The (Creation)	Draws the servant near to God.	Tranquillity	Pray for self and others to advance on the spiritual path.
90 Protector, The (Creation)	Repels those things which are harmful; prohibits and suppresses.	Self-Restraint	Provide material and spiritual richness to satisfy needs of the needy so they may repel those things which are harmful.
10 Proud, The (Self)	Everything less; only God has majesty and glory.	Aspiration	Self-centered, egotistical, haughty, arrogant, frail—we are nothing in comparison to God.
17 Provider, The (Humanity)	Creates means of sustenance as well as need for it and enjoyment of it; both knowledge based sustenance and material based.	Moral Reasonableness	Use speech to direct others to the Straight Path.
91 Punisher, The (Creation)	Secondary cause of what is harmful.	Self-Restraint	Suffering pain in our relationships.
40 Reckoner, The (Humanity)	God is the cause of being, continuation and perfection.	Thankfulness/ Generosity	Manage well God's blessings in relations with others; life is temporary.

B: List of the Translation of the 99 Most Beautiful Names with the Order, Division and Summary Description of Role in Theoethics, Psychoethics and Socioethics

Translation	Theoethics	Psychoethics	Socioethics
80 Repentance, The Acceptor of (Humanity)	Accepts repentance.	Repentance	Encourage self and others to repentance.
64 Resourceful, The (Self)	God lacks nothing.	Contentment	Be resourceful in relations with others.
59 Restorer, The (Creation)	Restores creation.	Moderation	Remember and recall for others the last creation on the Day of Judgment.
49 Resurrector, The (Creation)	Raising the dead; creation stage by stage revealing what is in people's hearts.	Piety	Teach knowledge and give life; plant here and reap in Hereafter; stages of creation.
88 Rich, The (Self)	God is not dependent on anything for essence or qualities; complete independence means richness.	Remembrance	Seek out the richness of God in relations with others.
98 Right in Guidance, The (Creation)	God is the right in guidance and the best of teachers leading towards the Straight Path and salvation.	Self-Restraint	Help teach others about the Straight Path.
63 Self-Existing, The (Self)	God requires nothing to exist.	Contentment	Detach self from everything but God in relations with others to be more objective.
13 Shaper of Unique Beauty, The (Creation)	Creates shapes of unique beauty.	Resolve	Create relationships of unique beauty with others.
61 Slayer, The (Creation)	Brings death into being.	Moderation	Die to your idol/ego self so that you relate to others through the heart.
3 Sovereign, The (Self)	God is independent of everything; powerful.	Aspiration	Develop sovereignty over the self through reason in relating to others.

B: List of the Translation of the 99 Most Beautiful Names with the Order, Division and Summary Description of Role in Theoethics, Psychoethics and Socioethics

Translation	Theoethics	Psychoethics	Socioethics
53 Strong, The (Self)	Perfect power; overcomes all opposition; unconditional strength.	Contentment	Be strong enough to overcome worldly temptations and help others do the same.
15 Subduer, The (Self)	Breaks back of His enemies.	Aspiration	Subdue, humiliate, kill the enemies within and without so our relationships with others are in harmony.
30 Subtle, The (Self)	Gentleness in action; delicacy of perception; knows hidden and manifest.	Self-Examination	Be gentle towards others.
35 Thankfulness, The Rewarder of (Humanity)	Unrestrained rewards for good deeds.	Thankfulness	Thankfulness by returning good with greater good.
52 Trustee, The (Humanity)	Everything is entrusted to God.	Trust	Be nature's trustee.
51 Truth, The (Self)	A cause of all that exists; existent by itself, does not change, has no beginning nor end.	Truthfulness	Remembering that the self is false and only God is real in our relations with others.
66 Unique, The (Self)	The Unique cannot be separated into parts: unity in multiplicity.	Unity	Manifest perfection of character—everything is from the Essence of One.
45 Vast, The (Self)	Expansiveness of knowledge and charity; no end to God's knowledge; embraces and contains all things.	Truthfulness	Develop extensive, all-inclusive wisdom and disposition without envy or greed or fear of poverty in relationships with others.
43 Vigilant, The (Humanity)	Knows, observes, watches out for a given object so we not approach the forbidden.	Vigilance	Being vigilant to inner enemies in relations with others.

B: List of the Translation of the 99 Most Beautiful Names with the Order, Division and Summary Description of Role in Theoethics, Psychoethics and Socioethics

Translation	Theoethics	Psychoethics	Socioethics
46 Wise, The (Self)	Order in the universe and it will continue until the Day of Judgment.	Truthfulness	To manifest sublime knowledge only comes from knowing God and remembering this in your relations with others.
50 Witness, The (Humanity)	Sees the visible and invisible.	Vigilance	Be aware of the visible and invisible in our relations with others.

C: List of the Number Symbolism (East) of the 99 Most Beautiful Names, Translation, Transliteration, Quality, Number Sybmolism (West), Division and Elemental Properties

ABJADE	Translation	Transliteration	Quality	ABJADW	Division	EAFW
13	One, The	al-Aḥad	C	13	Self	EEF
14	Bestower, The	al-Wahhāb	H	14	Humanity	AAFF
14	Resourceful, The	al-Wājid	B	14	Self	EAFW
18	Living, The	al-Ḥayy	B	18	Self	EA
19	Unique, The	al-Wāḥid	B	19	Self	EEAF
20	Loving, The	al-Wadūd	Be	20	Humanity	EEAA
20	Guide, The	al-Hādī	H	20	Humanity	EAFF
37	First, The	al-Awwal	H	37	Self	EAF
46	Friend, The	al-Walī	H	46	Humanity	EAA
47	Governor, The	al-Wālī	H	47	Creation	EAAF
48	Noble, The	al-Mājid	B	48	Self	EFFW
55	Prayer, The Responder to	al-Mujīb	H	55	Humanity	AAFW
56	Beginner, The	al-Mubdi'	H	56	Creation	EAAF
57	Glorious, The	al-Majīd	B	57	Self	EAFW
62	Praised, The	al-Ḥamīd	B	62	Self	EEAF
62	Hidden, The	al-Bāṭin	H	62	Self	AAFF
66	Trustee, The	al-Wakīl	B	66	Humanity	EAAW
68	Arbiter, The	al-Ḥakam	C	68	Self	EFW
68	Life-Giver, The	al-Muḥyī	H	68	Creation	EAAF
72	Expander, The	al-Bāsiṭ	B	312	Creation	EAFW
73	Majestic, The	al-Jalīl	C	73	Self	EEEA
78	Wise, The	al-Ḥakīm	B	78	Self	EAFW
80	Reckoner, The	al-Ḥasīb	B	320	Humanity	EAAW
86	Originator, The	al-Badī'	B	86	Self	EEAA
88	Forebearer, The	al-Ḥalīm	B	88	Humanity	EEAF
90	Sovereign, The	al-Malik	C	90	Self	EFW
94	Incomparable, The	al-'Aẓiz	C	94	Self	EAWW
104	Just, The	al-'Adl	C	104	Self	EEE
108	Truth, The	al-Ḥaqq	C	108	Self	EW
110	Highest, The	al-'Alī	C	110	Self	EEA
113	Everlasting, The	al-Bāqī	H	113	Self	AAFW
114	Gatherer, The	al-Jamī'	B	114	Creation	EFFW
116	Strong, The	al-Qawī	H	116	Self	AAW
117	Honorer, The	al-Mu'izz	C	117	Creation	EFW

C: List of the Number Symbolism (East) of the 99 Most Beautiful Names, Translation, Transliteration, Quality, Number Sybmolism (West), Division and Elemental Properties

ABJADE	Translation	Transliteration	Quality	ABJADW	Division	EAFW
124	Restorer, The	al-Mu'īd	B	124	Creation	EEAF
129	Subtle, The	al-Laṭīf	H	129	Self	EAFF
131	Flawless, The	al-Salām	H	371	Self	EFFF
134	Eternal, The	al-Ṣamad	H	104	Self	EAF
136	Faith, The Giver of	al-Mu'min	H	136	Humanity	AAFF
137	Vast, The	al-Wāsi'	B	377	Self	EAFW
145	Guardian, The	al-Muhaymin	H	145	Humanity	AAFFF
148	Appraiser, The	al-Muḥṣī	H	118	Creation	EAAF
150	Knower, The	al-'Alīm	B	150	Self	EEAF
156	Self-Existing, The	al-Qayyūm	H	156	Self	AAFW
156	Pardoner, The	al--'Afū	H	156	Humanity	EAF
161	Protector, The	al-Māni'	H	161	Creation	EAFF
170	Holy, The	al-Quddūs	C	410	Self	EAWW
180	All-Hearing, The	al-Samī'	H	420	Self	EAFF
184	Promoter, The	al-Muqaddim	C	184	Creation	EFFW
201	Creator of the Beneficial	al-Nāfi'	H	201	Creation	EAFF
202	Goodness, The Source of All	al-Barr	B	202	Self	EA
206	Compeller, The	al-Jabbār	B	206	Creation	EAFW
209	Equitable, The	al-Muqsiṭ	B	449	Creation	FFWW
212	King of Absolute Sovereignty	Mālik al-Mulk	B	212	Creation	EEEFFF-FFFWW
213	Maker of Perfect Harmony	al-Bāri'	H	213	Creation	EAAF
232	Great, The	al-Kabīr	B	232	Self	EAAW
256	Light, The	al-Nūr	H	256	Self	EAA
258	Compassionate, The	al-Raḥīm	B	258	Humanity	EEAF
270	Generous, The	al-Karīm	B	270	Humanity	EAFW
286	Clement, The	al-Ra'ūf	H	286	Humanity	EAF
298	Patient, The	al-Ṣabur	H	268	Humanity	EAAA
298	Merciful, The	al-Raḥmān	B	298	Humanity	EEAF
302	All-Seeing, The	al-Baṣīr	H	272	Self	EAAA
305	Able, The	al-Qādir	C	305	Self	EEFW
306	Subduer, The	al-Qahhār	B	306	Self	EFFW
308	Provider, The	al-Razzāq	C	308	Humanity	EFWW
312	Vigilant, The	al-Raqīb	B	312	Humanity	EAAW
319	Witness, The	al-Shahīd	H	1019	Humanity	EAFF
336	Shaper of Unique Beauty, The	al-Muṣawwir	H	306	Creation	EAAF

C: List of the Number Symbolism (East) of the 99 Most Beautiful Names, Translation, Transliteration, Quality, Number Sybmolism (West), Division and Elemental Properties

ABJADE	Translation	Transliteration	Quality	ABJADW	Division	EAFW
351	Exalter, The	al-Rāfi‘	B	351	Creation	EEFF
409	Repentance, The	al-Tawwāb	H	409	Humanity	AAAF
489	Opener, The	al-Fattāḥ	H	489	Humanity	EAFF
490	Slayer, The	al-Mumīt	H	490	Creation	AAFF
500	Firm, The	al-Matīin	H	500	Self	AAAF
514	Right in Guidance	al-Rashīd	B	1214	Creation	EEAF
526	Thankfulness, Rewarder of	al-Shakūr	B	1226	Humanity	EAFW
550	Maintainer, The	al-Muqīt	H	550	Humanity	AAFW
551	Exalted, The	al-Muta‘ālī	H	551	Self	EEAAFF
573	Resurrector, The	al-Bā‘ith	B	573	Creation	EAFW
630	Avenger, The	al-Muntaqim	H	630	Humanity	AAFFW
662	Proud, The	al-Mutakabbir	H	662	Self	EAAFW
707	Inheritor, The	al-Wārith	B	707	Creation	EAFW
731	Creator, The	al-Khāliq	C	731	Creation	EEFW
744	Powerful, The	al-Muqtadir	C	744	Creation	EEAFW
770	Dishonorer, The	al-Mudhill	H	770	Creation	EFF
801	Last, The	al-Ākhir	C	801	Self	EEF
812	Aware, The	al-Khabīr	B	812	Self	EEAA
846	Postponer, The	al-Mu’akhkhir	B	846	Creation	EEAF
903	Constrictor, The	al-Qābiḍ	H	193	Creation	AAFW
998	Preserver, The	al-Ḥafīẓ	Ba	898	Creation	EAFW
1001	Punisher, The	al-Ḍārr	H	291	Creation	EAF
1020	Magnificent, The	al-‘Aẓīm	B	920	Self	EAFW
1060	Rich, The	al-Ghanī	H	960	Self	EAA
1100	Lord of Majesty, Generosity	Dhu ’l-Jalāl wa ’l-Ikrām	H	1100	Self	EEEEEAA-AAFFFF-WW
1100	Enricher, The	al-Mughnī	H	1000	Humanity	EAAF
1106	Manifest, The	al-Zahīr	B	1006	Self	FFWW
1181	Forgiver, The	al-Ghaffār	B	1181	Humanity	EEFF
1186	Concealer of Faults, The	al-Ghafūr	B	1186	Humanity	EEAF
1481	Abaser, The	al-Khafīḍ	H	771	Creation	EAFF

D. List of the Quality of the 99 Most Beautiful Names, Translation, Transliteration, Number Symbolism (West and East), Divisions and Elemental Properties

Quality	Translation	Transliteration	ABJAD	W/E	Division	EAFW
B	Compassionate, The	al-Raḥīm	258	258	Humanity	EEAF
B	Compeller, The	al-Jabbār	206	206	Creation	EAFW
B	Forgiver, The	al-Ghaffār	1181	1181	Humanity	EEFF
B	Subduer, The	al-Qahhār	306	306	Self	EFFW
B	Knower, The	al-'Alīm	150	150	Self	EEAF
B	Expander, The	al-Bāsiṭ	312	72	Creation	EAFW
B	Exalter, The	al-Rāfi'	351	351	Creation	EEFF
B	Aware, The	al-Khabīr	812	812	Self	EEAA
B	Forebearing, The	al-Ḥalīm	88	88	Humanity	EEAF
B	Magnificent, The	al-'Aẓīm	920	1020	Self	
	Concealer of					EAFW
B	Faults, The	al-Ghafūr	1186	1186	Humanity	
	Thankfulness,					EEAF
B	Rewarder of	al-Shakūr	1226	526	Humanity	EAFW
B	Great, The	al-Kabīr	232	232	Self	EAAW
B	Reckoner, The	al-Ḥasīb	320	80	Humanity	EAAW
B	Generous, The	al-Karīm	270	270	Humanity	EAFW
B	Vigilant, The	al-Raqīb	312	312	Humanity	EAAW
B	Vast, The	al-Wāsi'	377	137	Self	EAFW
B	Wise, The	al-Ḥakīm	78	78	Self	EAFW
B	Loving, The	al-Wadūd	20	20	Humanity	EEAA
B	Glorious, The	al-Mājid	57	57	Self	EAFW
B	Resurrector, The	al-Bā'ith	573	573	Creation	EAFW
B	Trustee, The	al-Wakiil	66	66	Humanity	EAAW
B	Praised, The	al-Ḥamīd	62	62	Self	EEAF
B	Restorer, The	al-Mu'īd	124	124	Creation	EEAF
B	Living, The	al-Ḥayy	18	18	Self	EA
B	Resourceful, The	al-Wajīd	14	14	Self	EAFW
B	Noble, The	al-Majīd	48	48	Self	EFFW
B	Unique, The	al-Wāḥid	19	19	Self	EEAF
B	Postponer, The	al-Mu'akhkhir	846	846	Creation	EEAF
B	Manifest, The	al-Ẓahir	1006	1106	Self	FFWW
	Goodness, Source					
B	of All, The	al-Barr	202	202	Self	EA
	King of Absolute					EEEFF
B	Sovereignty	Mālik al-Mulk	449	209	Creation	FFWW
B	Equitable, The	al-Muqsiṭ	114	114	Creation	FFWW
B	Gatherer, The	al-Jāmi'	86	86	Creation	EFFW
B	Originator, The	al-Badī'	707	707	Self	EEAA

D. List of the Quality of the 99 Most Beautiful Names, Translation, Transliteration, Number Symbolism (West and East), Divisions and Elemental Properties

Quality	Translation	Transliteration	ABJAD W/E		Division	EAFW
B	Inheritor, The	al-Wārith	707	707	Creation	EAFW
B	Right in Guidance, The	al-Rashīd	1214	514	Creation	EEAF
C	Preserver, The	al-Ḥafīẓ	898	998	Cretion	EAFW
C	Merciful, The	al-Raḥmān	298	298	Humanity	EEAF
C	Sovereign, The	al-Malik	90	90	Self	EFW
C	Holy, The	al-Quddūs	410	170	Self	EAWW
C	Incomparable, The	al-ʻAzīz	94	94	Self	EAWW
C	Creator, The	al-Khāliq	731	731	Creqtion	EEFW
C	Provider, The	al-Razzāq	308	308	Humanity	EFWW
C	Honorer, The	al-Muʻizz	117	117	Creation	EFW
C	Arbiter, The	al-Ḥakam	68	68	Self	EFW
C	Just, The	al-ʻAdl	104	104	Self	EEE
C	Highest, The	al-ʻAlī	110	110	Self	EEA
C	Majestic, The	al-Jalīl	73	73	Self	EEEA
C	Truth, The	al-Ḥaqq	108	108	Self	EW
C	One, The	al-Aḥad	13	13	Self	EEF
C	Able, The	al-Qādir	305	305	Self	EEFW
C	Powerful, The	al-Muqtadir	744	744	Creation	EEAFW
C	Promoter, The	al-Muqaddim	184	184	Creation	EFFW
H	Last, The	al-Ākhir	801	801	Self	EEF
H	Flawless, The	al-Salām	371	131	Self	EFFF
H	Faith, The Giver of	al-Mu'min	136	136	Humanity	AAFF
H	Guardian, The	al-Muhaymin	145	145	Humanity	AAFFF
H	Proud, The	al-Mutakabbir	662	662	Self	EAAFW
H	Maker of Perfect Harmony	al-Bāri'	213	213	Creation	EAAF
H	Shaper of Unique Beauty	al-Muṣawwir	306	336	Creation	EAAF
H	Bestower, The	al-Wahhāb	14	14	Humanity	AAFF
H	Opener, The	al-Fattāḥ	489	489	Humanity	EAFF
H	Constrictor, The	al-Qabīd	193	903	Creation	AAFW
H	Abaser, The	al-Khafīḍ	771	1481	Creation	EAFF
H	Dishonorer, The	al-Mudhill	770	770	Creation	EFF
H	All-Hearing, The	al-Samīʻ	420	180	Self	EAFF
H	All-Seeing, The	al-Baṣīr	272	302	Self	EAAA
H	Subtle, The	al-Laṭif	129	129	Self	EAFF
H	Maintainer, The	al-Muqīt	55	55	Humanity	AAFW

D. List of the Quality of the 99 Most Beautiful Names, Translation, Transliteration, Number Symbolism (West and East), Divisions and Elemental Properties

Quality	Translation	Transliteration	ABJAD W	E	Division	EAFW
H	Prayer, Responder to, The	al-Mujīb	55	55	Humanity	AAFW
H	Witness, The	al-Shāhid	1019	319	Humanity	EAFF
H	Strong, The	al-Qawī	116	116	Self	AAW
H	Firm, The	al-Matīn	500	500	Self	AAAF
H	Friend, The	al-Walī	46	46	Humanity	EAA
H	Appraiser, The	al-Muḥṣī	118	148	Creation	EAAF
H	Beginner, The	al-Mubdi'	56	56	Creation	EAAF
H	Life-Giver, The	al-Muḥyī	68	68	Creation	EAAF
H	Self-Existing, The	al-Qayyūm	156	156	Self	AAFW
H	Eternal, The	al-Ṣamad	104	134	Self	EAF
H	First, The	al-Awwal	37	37	Self	EAF
H	Hidden, The	al-Bāṭin	62	62	Self	AAFF
H	Governor, The	al-Wālī	47	47	Creation	EAAF
H	Exalted, The	al-Muta'ālī	551	551	Self	EEAAFF
H	Repentance, The	al-Tawwāb	409	409	Humanity	AAAF
H	Avenger, The	al-Muntaqim	630	630	Humanity	AAFFW
H	Pardoner, The	al-'Afū	156	156	Humanity	EAF
H	Clement, The	al-Ra'ūf	286	286	Humanity	EAF
H	Lord of Majesty, Generosity	Dhū 'l-Jalāl wa 'l-Ikrām				EEEEE AAAAF FFF-FWW
H	Rich, The	al-Ghanī	1100	1100	Self	EAA
H	Enricher, The	al-Mughnī	960	1060	Self	EAAF
H	Protector, The	al-Māni'	1000	1100	Humanity	EAFF
H	Punisher, The	al-Ḍārr	161	161	Creation	EAF
H	Creator of the Beneficial, The	al-Nāfi'	291	1001	Creation	EAFF
H	Light, The	al-Nūr	201	201	Creation	EAA
H	Everlasting, The	al-Bāqī	256	256	Self	AAFW
H	Patient, The	al-Ṣabur	113	113	Self	EAAA
H	Guide, The	al-Hādī	268	298	Humanity	EAFF
H	Slayer, The	al-Mumīt	20	20	Humanity	AAFF
			490	490	Creation	

E: List of the Translation of the 99 Most Beautiful Names, Their Letters and Number Symbolism (East) and Their Elemental Properties

Translation	Transliteration	ABJADE	Letters East	EAFW
Abaser, The	al-Khāfiḍ	1481	600+1+80+800	EAFF
Able, The	al-Qādir	305	100+1+4+200	EEFW
All-Hearing, The	al-Samī‘	180	60+40+10+70	EAFF
All-Seeing, The	al-Baṣīr	302	2+90+10+200	EAAA
Appraiser, The	al-Muḥṣī	148	40+8+90+10	EAAF
Arbiter, The	al-Ḥakam	68	8+20+40	EFW
Avenger, The	al-Muntaqim	630	40+50+400+100+40	AAFFW
Aware, The	al-Khabīr	812	600+2+10+200	EEAA
Beginner, The	al-Mubdi’	56	40+2+4+10	EAAF
Bestower, The	al-Wahhāb	14	6+5+1+2	AAFF
Clement, The	al-Ra’ūf	286	200+6+80	EAF
Compassionate, The	al-Raḥīm	258	200+8+10+40	EEAF
Compeller, The	al-Jabbār	206	3+2+1+200	EAFW
Concealer of Faults, The	al-Ghafūr	1186	900+80+6+200	EEAF
Constrictor, The	al-Qābid	903	100+1+2+800	AAFW
Creator of the Beneficial	al-Nāfi‘	201	50+1+80+70	EAFF
Punisher, The	al-Ḍārr	1001	800+1+200	EAF
Creator, The	al-Khāliq	731	600+30+1+100	EEFW
Dishonorer, The	al-Mudhill	770	40+700+30	EFF
Enricher, The	al-Mughnī	1100	40+1000+50+10	EAAF
Equitable, The	al-Muqsiṭ	209	40+100+60+9	FFWW
Eternal, The	al-Ṣamad	134	90+40+4	EAF
Everlasting, The	al-Bāqī	113	2+1+100+10	AAFW
Exalted, The	al-Muta‘ālī	551	40+400+70+1+30+10	EEAAFF
Exalter, The	al-Rāfi‘	351	200+1+80+70	EEFF
Expander, The	al-Bāsiṭ	72	2+1+60+9	EAFW
Faith, The Giver of	al-Mu’min	136	40+6+40+50	AAFF
Firm, The	al-Matīn	500	40+400+10+50	AAAF
First, The	al-Awwal	37	1+6+30	EAF
Flawless, The	al-Salām	131	60+30+1+40	EFFF
Forebearing, The	al-Ḥalīm	88	8+30+10+40	EEAF
Forgiver, The	al-Ghaffār	1181	900+80+1+200	EEFF
Friend, The	al-Walī	46	6+1+30+10	EAA
Gatherer, The	al-Jāmi‘	114	3+1+40+70	EFFW
Generous, The	al-Karīm	270	20+200+10+40	EAFW
Glorious, The	al-Majīd	57	40+3+10+4	EAFW

E: List of the Translation of the 99 Most Beautiful Names, Their Letters and Number Symbolism (East) and Their Elemental Properties

Translation	Transliteration	ABJADE	Letters East	EAFW
Goodness, Source of All, The	al-Barr	202	2+200	EA
Governor, The	al-Wālī	47	6+1+30+10	EAAF
Great, The	al-Kabīr	232	20+2+10+200	EAAW
Guardian, The	al-Muhaymin	145	40+5+10+40+50	AAFFF
Guide, The	al-Hādī	20	5+1+4+10	EAFF
Hidden, The	al-Bāṭin	62	2+1+9+50	AAFF
Highest, The	al-'Alī	110	70+30+10	EEA
Holy, The	al-Quddūs	170	100+4+6+60	EAWW
Honorer, The	al-Mu'izz	117	40+70+7	EFW
Incomparable, The	al-'Azīz	94	70+7+10+7	EAWW
Inheritor, The	al-Wārith	707	6+1+200+500	EAFW
Just, The	al-'Adl	104	70+4+30	EEE
King of Absolute Sovereignty	Mālik al-Mulk	212	40+1+30+20+1+30+40+30+20	EEEFFF-FWW
Knower, The	al-'Alīm	150	70+30+10+40	EEAF
Last, The	al-Ākhir	801	1+600+200	EEF
Life-Giver, The	al-Muḥyī	68	40+8+10+10	EAAF
Light, The	al-Nūr	256	50+6+200	EAA
Living, The	al-Ḥayy	18	8+10	EA
Lord of Majesty, Generosity	Dhū 'l-Jalāl wa 'l-Ikrām	1100	700+6+1+30+3+30+1+30+6+1+30+1+20+200+1+40	EEEEEAAAAFFFFFWW
Loving, The	al-Wadūd	20	6+4+6+4	EEAA
Magnificent, The	al-'Aẓīm	1020	70+900+10+40	EAFW
Maintainer, The	al-Muqīt	550	40+100+10+400	AAFW
Majestic, The	al-Jalīl	73	3+30+10+30	EEEA
Maker of Perfect Harmony, The	al-Bāri'	213	2+1+200+10	EAAF
Manifest, The	al-Ẓahir	1106	900+1+5+200	FFWW
Merciful, The	al-Raḥmān	298	200+8+40+50	EEAF
Noble, The	al-Majīd	48	40+1+3+4	EFFW
One, The	al-Aḥad	13	1+8+4	EEF
Opener, The	al-Fattāḥ	489	80+400+1+8	EAFF
Originator, The	al-Badī'	86	2+4+10+70	EEAA
Pardoner, The	al-'Afū	156	70+80+6	EAF
Patient, The	al-Ṣabur	298	90+2+6+200	EAAA
Postponer, The	al-Mu'akhkhir	846	40+6+600+200	EEAF
Powerful, The	al-Muqtadir	744	40+100+400+4+200	EEAFW
Praised, The	al-Ḥamīd	62	8+40+10+4	EEAF

E: List of the Translation of the 99 Most Beautiful Names, Their Letters and Number Symbolism (East) and Their Elemental Properties

Translation	Transliteration	ABJADE	Letters East	EAFW
Prayer, The Responder to	al-Mujīb	55	40+3+10+2	AAFW
Preserver, The	al-Ḥafiẓ	998	8+80+10+900	EAFW
Promoter, The	al-Muqaddim	184	40+100+4+40	EFFW
Protector, The	al-Māni‘	161	40+1+50+70	EAFF
Proud, The	al-Mutakabbir	662	40+400+20+2+200	EAAFW
Provider, The	al-Razzāq	308	200+7+1+100	EFWW
Reckoner, The	al-Ḥasīb	80	8+60+10+2	EAAW
Repentance, The	al-Tawwāb	409	400+6+1+2	AAAF
Resourceful, The	al-Wajīd	14	6+1+3+4	EAFW
Restorer, The	al-Mu‘īd	124	40+70+10+4	EEAF
Resurrector, The	al-Ba‘ith	573	2+1+70+500	EAFW
Rich, The	al-Ghanīi	1060	1000+50+10	EAA
Right in Guidance, The	al-Rashīd	514	200+300+10+4	EEAF
Self-Existing, The	al-Qayyūm	156	100+10+6+40	AAFW
Shaper of Unique Beauty	al-Muṣawwir	336	40+90+6+200	EAAF
Slayer, The	al-Mumīt	490	40+40+10+400	AAFF
Sovereign, The	al-Malik	90	40+30+20	EFW
Strong, The	al-Qawī	116	100+6+10	AAW
Subduer, The	al-Qāhhar	306	100+5+1+200	EFFW
Subtle, The	al-Laṭīf	129	30+9+10+80	EAFF
Thankfulness, The Rewarder of	al-Shakūr	526	300+20+6+200	EAFW
Trustee, The	al-Wakīl	66	6+20+10+30	EAAW
Truth, The	al-Ḥaqq	108	8+100	EW
Unique, The	al-Wāḥid	19	6+1+8+4	EEAF
Vast, The	al-Wāsi‘	137	6+1+60+70	EAFW
Vigilant, The	al-Raqīb	312	200+100+10+2	EAAW
Wise, The	al-Ḥakīm	78	8+20+10+40	EAFW
Witness, The	al-Shāhid	319	300+5+10+4	EAFF

F: List of the Translation of the 99 Most Beautiful Names, Their Letters and Number Symbolism (West) and Their Elemental Properties

Translation	Transliteration	ABJADW	Letters WEST	EAFW
Abaser, The	al-Khāfiḍ	771	600+1+80+90	EAFF
Able, The	al-Qādir	305	100+1+4+200	EEFW
All-Hearing, The	al-Samī'	420	300+40+10+70	EAFF
All-Seeing, The	al-Baṣīr	272	2+60+10+200	EAAA
Appraiser, The	al-Muḥṣī	118	40+8+60+10	EAAF
Arbiter, The	al-Ḥakam	68	8+20+40	EFW
Avenger, The	al-Muntaqim	630	40+50+400+100+40	AAFFW
Aware, The	al-Khabīr	812	600+2+10+200	EEAA
Beginner, The	al-Mubdi'	56	40+2+4+10	EAAF
Bestower, The	al-Wahhāb	14	6+5+1+2	AAFF
Clement, The	al-Ra'ūf	286	200+6+80	EAF
Compassionate, The	al-Raḥīm	258	200+8+10+40	EEAF
Compeller, The	al-Jabbār	206	3+2+1+200	EAFW
Concealer of Faults, The	al-Ghafūr	1186	900+80+6+200	EEAF
Constrictor, The	al-Qābid	903	100+1+2+800	AAFW
Creator of the Beneficial	al-Nāfi'	201	50+1+80+70	EAFF
Punisher, The	al-Ḍārr	291	90+1+200	EAF
Creator, The	al-Khāliq	731	600+30+1+100	EEFW
Dishonorer, The	al-Mudhill	770	40+700+30	EFF
Enricher, The	al-Mughnī	1000	40+900+50+10	EAAF
Equitable, The	al-Muqsiṭ	449	40+100+300+9	FFWW
Eternal, The	al-Ṣamad	104	60+40+4	EAF
Everlasting, The	al-Bāqī	113	2+1+100+10	AAFW
Exalted, The	al-Muta'ālī	551	40+400+70+1+30+10	EEAAFF
Exalter, The	al-Rāfi'	351	200+1+80+70	EEFF
Expander, The	al-Bāsiṭ	312	2+1+300+9	EAFW
Faith, The Giver of	al-Mu'min	136	40+6+40+50	AAFF
Firm, The	al-Matīn	500	40+400+10+50	AAAF
First, The	al-Awwal	37	1+6+30	EAF
Flawless, The	al-Salām	371	300+30+1+40	EFFF
Forebearing, The	al-Ḥalīm	88	8+30+10+40	EEAF
Forgiver, The	al-Ghaffār	1181	900+80+1+200	EEFF
Friend, The	al-Walī	46	6+1+30+10	EAA
Gatherer, The	al-Jāmi'	114	3+1+40+70	EFFW
Generous, The	al-Karīm	270	20+200+10+40	EAFW
Glorious, The	al-Majīd	57	40+3+10+4	EAFW

F: List of the Translation of the 99 Most Beautiful Names, Their Letters and Number Symbolism (West) and Their Elemental Properties

Translation	Transliteration	ABJADW	Letters WEST	EAFW
Goodness, The Source of All	al-Barr	202	2+200	EA
Governor, The	al-Wālī	47	6+1+30+10	EAAF
Great, The	al-Kabīr	232	20+2+10+200	EAAW
Guardian, The	al-Muhaymin	145	40+5+10+40+50	AAFFF
Guide, The	al-Hādī	20	5+1+4+10	EAFF
Hidden, The	al-Bāṭin	62	2+1+9+50	AAFF
Highest, The	al-'Alī	110	70+30+10	EEA
Holy, The	al-Quddūs	410	100+4+6+300	EAWW
Honorer, The	al-Mu'izz	117	40+70+7	EFW
Incomparable, The	al-'Azīz	94	70+7+10+7	EAWW
Inheritor, The	al-Wārith	707	6+1+200+500	EAFW
Just, The	al-'Adl	104	70+4+30	EEE
King of Absolute Sovereignty	Mālik al-Mulk	212	40+1+30+20+1+30+40+ 30+20	EEEFFF- FWW
Knower, The	al-'Alīm	150	70+30+10+40	EEAF
Last, The	al-Ākhir	801	1+600+200	EEF
Life-Giver, The	al-Muḥyī	68	40+8+10+10	EAAF
Light, The	al-Nūr	256	50+6+200	EAA
Living, The	al-Ḥayy	18	8+10	EA
Lord of Majesty, Generosity	Dhū 'l-Jalāl wa 'l-Ikrām	1100	700+6+1+30+3+30+1+30+ 6+1+30+1+20+200+1+40	EEEEEAAAA FFFFFWW
Loving, The	al-Wadūd	20	6+4+6+4	EEAA
Magnificent, The	al-'Aẓīm	920	70+800+10+40	EAFW
Maintainer, The	al-Muqīt	550	40+100+10+400	AAFW
Majestic, The	al-Jalīl	73	3+30+10+30	EEEA
Maker of Perfect Harmony	al-Bāri'	213	2+1+200+10	EAAF
Manifest, The	al-Ẓahir	1006	800+1+5+200	FFWW
Merciful, The	al-Raḥmān	298	200+8+40+50	EEAF
Noble, The	al-Majīd	48	40+1+3+4	EFFW
One, The	al-Aḥad	13	1+8+4	EEF
Opener, The	al-Fattāḥ	489	80+400+1+8	EAFF
Originator, The	al-Badī'	86	2+4+10+70	EEAA
Pardoner, The	al-'Afū	156	70+80+6	EAF
Patient, The	al-Ṣabur	268	60+2+6+200	EAAA
Postponer, The	al-Mu'akhkhir	846	40+6+600+200	EEAF
Powerful, The	al-Muqtadir	744	40+100+400+4+200	EEAFW
Praised, The	al-Ḥamīd	62	8+40+10+4	EEAF

F: List of the Translation of the 99 Most Beautiful Names, Their Letters and Number Symbolism (West) and Their Elemental Properties

TRANSLATION	TRANSLITERATION	ABJADW	LETTERS WEST	EAFW
Prayer, The Responder to	al-Mujīb	55	40+3+10+2	AAFW
Preserver, The	al-Ḥafīẓ	898	8+80+10+800	EAFW
Promoter, The	al-Muqaddim	184	40+100+4+40	EFFW
Protector, The	al-Māni'	161	40+1+50+70	EAFF
Proud, The	al-Mutakabbir	662	40+400+20+2+200	EAAFW
Provider, The	al-Razzāq	308	200+7+1+100	EFWW
Reckoner, The	al-Ḥasīb	320	8+300+10+2	EAAW
Repentance, The	al-Tawwāb	409	400+6+1+2	AAAF
Resourceful, The	al-Wajīd	14	6+1+3+4	EAFW
Restorer, The	al-Mu'īd	124	40+70+10+4	EEAF
Resurrector, The	al-Ba'ith	573	2+1+70+500	EAFW
Rich, The	al-Ghanīi	960	900+50+10	EAA
Right in Guidance, The	al-Rashīd	1214	200+1000+10+4	EEAF
Self-Existing, The	al-Qayyūm	156	100+10+6+40	AAFW
Shaper of Unique Beauty	al-Muṣawwir	306	40+60+6+200	EAAF
Slayer, The	al-Mumīt	490	40+40+10+400	AAFF
Sovereign, The	al-Malik	90	40+30+20	EFW
Strong, The	al-Qawī	116	100+6+10	AAW
Subduer, The	al-Qāhhar	306	100+5+1+200	EFFW
Subtle, The	al-Laṭīf	129	30+9+10+80	EAFF
Thankfulness, The Rewarder of	al-Shakūr	1226	1000+20+6+200	EAFW
Trustee, The	al-Wakīl	66	6+20+10+30	EAAW
Truth, The	al-Ḥaqq	108	8+100	EW
Unique, The	al-Wāḥid	19	6+1+8+4	EEAF
Vast, The	al-Wāsi'	377	6+1+300+70	EAFW
Vigilant, The	al-Raqīb	312	200+100+10+2	EAAW
Wise, The	al-Ḥakīm	78	8+20+10+40	EAFW
Witness, The	al-Shāhid	1019	1000+5+10+4	EAFF

G: List of the Transliteration of the 99 Most Beautiful Names, Their Invocation (dhikr) with an Index to Special Properties*

Transliteration	Order	Translation	Invocation
al-'Adl	29	Just, The	Write yā 'Adl on a piece of bread on Thursday night and eat the bread and people may obey you.
Al-'Afu	82	Pardoner, The	Repeat yā 'Afu frequently and your wrong doings should be forgiven.
al-Aḥad	67	One, The	
al-Ākhir	74	Last, The	Those who recite yā Ākhir frequently should lead a good life and have a good end at the time of death.
al-'Alī	36	Highest, The	If your faith is low and you repeat yā 'Alī frequently, your faith should be raised and your destiny opened.
al- 'Alīm	19	Knower, The	Repeat yā 'Alīm 100 times after every prescribed prayer and God should give you spiritual unveiling or intuition (*kashf*). If you want to know about hidden work, you should go down in prostration on Friday night and say yā 'Alīm 100 times and sleep there. If you frequently recite yā 'Alīm, God may illuminate your heart and reveal Divine Light. If you desire something, you should perform ablution, go to a forest, face the direction of prayer (*qiblah*), offer a two cycle prayer and then recite yā 'Alīm 1000 times and it may be given.
al-Awwal	73	First, The	Recite yā Awwal 40 times on Thursday nights and your needs should be fulfilled.
al-'Aẓim	33	Magnificent, The	Recite yā 'Aẓim frequently and you may develop respect among people.
al-'Azīz	8	Incomparable, The	If you recite yā 'Azīz for forty days between the prescribed and recommended dawn prescribed prayer, you should not be needy.
al-Bā'ith	49	Resurrector, The	Frequently recite yā Bā'ith 100 times and you should gain fear of God.
al-Badī'	95	Originator, The	Repeat yā Badī' 1000 times by saying, "*Yā Badī' as-samavatī wa 'l-arḍ*," "Oh Originator of the heavens and the earth," and your troubles may disappear.
al- Bāqī	96	Everlasting, The	Recite yā Bāqī on Thursday night and you should be free of difficulties.
al-Bāri'	12	Maker of Perfect Harmony, The	Recite ya Bāri' frequently and your hard work should become easy.
al-Barr	79	Goodness, The Source of All	Repeat ya Barr frequently and one should be blessed and free from misfortune.

* Remembering God (*dhikr Allah*) or invocation through the 99 Most Beautiful Names is based on Naghsbandi Dihlavi's *Jawahir al-khamseh* and other Sufi prayer books.

G: List of the Transliteration of the 99 Most Beautiful Names, Their Invocation (dhikr) with an Index to Special Properties

Transliteration	Order	Translation	Invocation
al-Baṣīr	27	All-Seeing, The	Recite yā Baṣīr 100 times after the Friday prescribed congregational prayer and God should give you esteem in the eyes of others.
al-Bāsiṭ	21	Expander, The	Recite yā Bāsiṭ 10 times after the dawn prescribed prayer with open hands, palms up and then rub your face with your hands and you should be freed of the need of others.
al-Bāṭin	76	Hidden, The	Recite yā Bāṭin 22 times each day and you should see the truth in things.
al-Ḍārr	91	Punisher, The	Whoever has been in the same state or condition for a long time and wants to get into a better state should repeat yā Ḍārr 100 times on Thursday nights to grow closer to God.
Dhū 'l-Jalāl wa 'l-Ikrām	85	Lord of Majesty and Generosity	Repeat yā Dhū 'l-Jalāl wa 'l-Ikrām frequently and you may develop esteem among people.
al-Fattāḥ	18	Opener, The	With hands on your chest, repeat yā Fattāḥ 70 times after the dawn prescribed prayer and your spiritual heart should then become free of rust and be opened, given victory over the idol/ego and purified.
al-Gaffār	14	Forgiver, The	Recite yā Gaffār 100 times after the Friday prescribed congregational prayer and your sins should be forgiven.
al-Ghafūr	34	Concealer of Faults, The	Whenever you suffer from a headache, fever or temporary despair and despondency, you should recite yā Ghafūr continuously and you may be relieved of your ailment.
al-Ghanī	88	Rich, The	Repeat yā Ghanī frequently and you may become contented and not covetous.
al-Hādī	94	Guide, The	Repeat yā Hādī frequently and you should gain spiritual knowledge.
al-Ḥafīẓ	38	Preserver, The	Recite yā Ḥafīẓ 16 times a day and you should be protected from calamities.
al-Ḥakam	28	Arbiter, The	If you recite yā Ḥakam on Thursday night in the middle of the night so frequently and continuously that you lose consciousness and faints, you may come to know the hidden meanings in things.
al-Ḥakīm	46	Wise, The	Recite yā Ḥakīm frequently and your difficulties in work should be overcome.
al-Ḥalīm	32	Forebearer, The	Write yā Ḥalīm on a piece of paper and put the paper wherever you plant something to preserve it from harm, disaster or calamity.
al-Ḥamīd	56	Praised, The	Repeat yā Ḥamīd frequently and you may be loved and praised.

G: List of the Transliteration of the 99 Most Beautiful Names, Their Invocation (dhikr) with an Index to Special Properties

Transliteration	Order	Translation	Invocation
al-Ḥaqq	51	Truth, The	One who recites yā Ḥaqq should find something lost.
al-Ḥasīb	40	Reckoner, The	Repeat yā Ḥasīb 70 times on Thursday during the day and night for seven days and nights and the 71st time say, "Allāh al-Ḥasīb," "God is my Reckoner," and you should be freed of the fear of being robbed, or the jealousy of another or being harmed or wronged.
al-Ḥayy	62	Living, The	Recite yā Ḥayy frequently and you may gain a long life. If you are sick, you may be cured.
al- Jabbār	9	Compeller, The	Frequently repeat yā Jabbār 21 times each time and you should not be compelled to do anything against your wishes and you should not be exposed to violence, severity or hardship.
al-Jalīl	41	Majestic, The	Write yā Jalīl on a piece of paper with saffron and musk ink. Wash the paper and put the liquid into a ceramic container. Drink from the earthen container and you may be revered among people.
al-Jāmi'	87	Gatherer, The	Repeat yā Jāmi' frequently to find things lost.
al-Kabīr	37	Great, The	Requently repeat yā Kabīr 100 times and you should develop esteem and respect among people.
al-Karīm	42	Generous, The	Recite yā Karīm frequently and you should have esteem in this world.
al-Khabīr	31	Aware, The	Recite yā Khabīr frequently and you should be quickly freed of a bad habit.
al-Khāfiḍ	22	Abaser, The	Fast for three days and on the fourth day, recite yā Khāfiḍ 70,000 times in a gathering and you should be free from harm by your enemy.
al-Khāliq	11	Creator, The	Recite yā Khāliq frequently at night and God may help you act for His sake.
al-Laṭīf	30	Subtle, The	If you have become poverty-stricken or lonely or wish a desire to be fulfilled or have become sick without anyone to care for you, recite yā Laṭīf 100 times while performing the prescribed ablution and your prayer may be heard.
al-Majīd	48	Glorious, The	Recite yā Majīd frequently and you should gain glory.
al-Mājid	65	Noble, The	Recite yā Mājid frequently and your heart may be enlightened.

G: List of the Transliteration of the 99 Most Beautiful Names, Their Invocation (dhikr) with an Index to Special Properties

Transliteration	Order	Translation	Invocation
Mālik al-Mulk	84	King of Absolute Sovereignty	Recite yā Mālik al-Mulk frequently and you should gain esteem among people.
al-Malik	3	Sovereign, The	Recite ya Malik frequently and you may be treated with respect by others.
al-Māni'	90	Protector, The	Repeat ya Māni' frequently and you should have a good family life. Frequently recite 20 times and God should subside your anger.
al-Matīn	54	Firm, The	Recite yā Matīn frequenlty if you have troubles and your troubles should disappear.
al-Mu'akhkhir	72	Postponer, The	Recite yā Mu'akhkhir 100 times frequently in your heart and only love of God should remain. No other love can enter.
al-Mubdi'	58	Beginner, The	Repeat ya Mubdi' and breathe towards someone who is about to lose something and that person should become free of danger.
al-Mudhill	25	Dishonorer, The	Recite yā Mudhill 75 times when you sense harm from a jealous person and you should be protected by God. If you go to prostration and say, "Oh God save me from the oppression of so and so..." and you should be safe.
al-Mughnī	89	Enricher, The	Recite yā Mughnī 1000 times every Friday and you should become self-sufficient.
al-Muhaymin	7	Guardian, The	Recite yā Muhaymin after the prescribed ablution 115 times and your inner being may be illuminated.
al-Muhsī	57	Appraiser, The	Recite yā Muhsī 100 times frequently and you should receive ease on the Day of Judgment.
al-Muḥyī	60	Life-Giver, The	If you are weighed down with a heavy burden and repeat yā Muḥyī 7 times a day, you should have your burden removed.
al-Mu'īd	59	Restorer, The	Repeat ya Mu'īd 70 times for someone away from his or her family and he or she should return safely.
al-Muizz	24	Honorer, The	Repeat yā Mu'izz 140 times after the evening prescribed prayer on Sunday and Thursday night and you should develop dignity in eyes of others and fear no one but God.
al-Mujīb	44	Prayer, The Responder to	Recite yā Mujīb frequently and supplicate and you should continue to have faith.
al-Mu'min	6	Faith, the Giver of	Recite yā Mu'min frequently and you should be freed from the harm of your idol/ego.

G: List of the Transliteration of the 99 Most Beautiful Names, Their Invocation (dhikr) with an Index to Special Properties

Transliteration	Order	Translation	Invocation
yā Mumīt	61	Slayer, The	Recite yā Mumīt frequently with your hands on your chest on falling asleep and you should be able to control your passions and destroy your enemy.
al-Muntaqim	81	Avenger, The	Repeat yā Mutaqim frequently and you should be victorious against your enemy.
al-Muqaddim	71	Promoter, The	Repeat yā Muqaddim on the battlefield or when you are afraid of being alone in a frightening place and no harm should come to you.
al-Muqī	39	Maintainer, The	If someone is ill-mannered. repeat yā Muqīt several times into a glass of water and give it to the person to drink and the person may develop good manners.
al-Muqsiṭ	86	Equitable, The	Repeat yā Muqsiṭ 100 times and you should be free from the harm of your idol/ego and you should attain your purpose.
al-Muqtadir	70	Powerful, The	Repeat yā Muqtadir frequently and you should become aware of the Truth.
al-Muṣawwir	13	Shaper of Unique Beauty, The	Recite yā Muṣawwir frequently and hard work should become easy.
al-Muta'ālī	78	Exalted, The	Repeat ya Muta'ālī frequently and you should gain the benevolence of God and difficulties should ease.
al-Mutakabbir	10	Proud, The	Begin every act with yā Mutakabbir and you may get your wish.
al-Nāfi'	92	Creator of the Beneficial, The	Repeat yā Nāfi' for four days as many times as you can and you should be able to avoid harm.
al-Nūr	93	Light, The	Repeat yā Nūr frequently and perhaps gain inner light. Recite yā Nūr 700 times on Thursday night and you may receive inner light. Recite Surah Nūr 7 times and yā Nūr 1000 times and you may gian light in your heart.
al-Qābiḍ	20	Constrictor, The	For forty days write yā Qābiḍ on a piece of bread and eat it and you should be safe from the punishment of the grave and from hunger.
al-Qādir	69	Able, The	Recite yā Qādir while washing each limb during the performance of the prescribed ablution and you should never fall into the grip of an oppressor and no enemy should harm you. If you face a difficulty and recite yā Qādir 41 times, God should free you from of that difficulty.

G: List of the Transliteration of the 99 Most Beautiful Names, Their Invocation (dhikr) with an Index to Special Properties

Transliteration	Order	Translation	Invocation
al-Qahhār	15	Subduer, The	If you recites yā Qahhār 100 times between the obligatory and recommended dawn prescribed prayer, you should be able to overcome your enemy. If you repeat yā Qahhār frequently, you should be able to conquer the desires of your attraction to pleasure system, gain inner peace and be freed from being wronged by another.
al-Qawī	53	Strong, The	If you cannot defeat an enemy and repeat yā Qawī frequently with the intention of not being harmed, you should be freed of any harm by your enemy.
al-Qayyūm	63	Self-Existing, The	Recite yā Qayyūm at the time of the dawn prescribed prayer and people may keep you as a friend.
al-Quddūs	4	Holy, The	If you recite yā Quddūs each day at sunset, your heart may expand.
al-Rāfi'	23	Exalter, The	Recite yā Rāfi' 100 times on Thursday and Sunday night and you should attain a higher sense of honor, richness and merit.
al-Raḥīm	2	Compassionate, The	Repeat yā Raḥīm 100 times after each dawn prrescribed prayer and everyone should become friendly towards you.
al-Raḥmān	1	Merciful, The	Repeat yā Raḥmān 100 times after each obligatory prayer and you should develop a good memory, keen awareness and be freed of a heavy heart.
al-Raqīb	43	Vigilant, The	Repat yā Raqīb 7 times for yourself, family and property to be under God's protection.
al-Rashīd	98	Right in Guidance, The	Repeat yā Rashīd 1000 times between the evening prescribed prayer and the night prescribed prayer and your troubles should clear up.
al-Ra'ūf	83	Clement, The	Repeat yā Ra'ūf frequently and you should be blessed by God and His people.
al-Razzāq	17	Provider, The	Standing and facing the direction of the prescribed prayer (*qiblah*), repeat yā Razzāq 10 times and then 10 times in the other three directions and you should not suffer poverty. Repeat 545 times and you should have your sustenance. Go into seclusion (*khalwat*) and repeat 1000 times and you should meet Khidr if your sustenance is permissible.
al-Ṣabur	99	Patient, The	Repeat yā Ṣabur 33 times and you should be rescued from troubles, difficulties and sorrow.

G: List of the Transliteration of the 99 Most Beautiful Names, Their Invocation (dhikr) with an Index to Special Properties

Transliteration	Order	Translation	Invocation
al-Salām	5	Flawless, The	Recite yā Salām 100 times to a sick person and he or she may regain health.
al-Ṣamad	68	Eternal, The	Repeat yā Ṣamad 1000 times and you may come to know the hidden meanings of things. If you recite yā Ṣamad 115 times at dawn or in the middle of the night while in prostration, you should never fall into the grip of an oppressor.
al-Samī'	26	All-Hearing, The	Recite yā Samī' 500 times after performing the noon obligatory prayer and God should give you your desire and your prayer should be heard.
al-Shahīd	50	Witness, The	Repeat yā Shahīd 21 times with your hand on the forehead of a rebellious child and the child may become obedient.
al-Shakūr	35	Thankfulness, The Rewarder of	If you have a heavy heart, repeat yā Shakūr 41 times into a glass of water and wash your face with that water and your heart should lighten up and you should be able to maintain your composure.
al-Tawwāb	80	Repentance, The Acceptor of	Repeat yā Tawwāb many times and your repentance should be accepted.
al-Wadūd	47	Loving, The	If there has been a quarrel between two people and one of the two repeats yā Wadūd 1000 times over food and gives the food to the other to eat, the disagreement may be resolved.
al-Wahhāb	16	Bestower, The	Repeat yā Wahhāb 7 times at midnight after supplication and your appeal may be answered. If you have a desire, or have been captured by an enemy or you cannot earn enough, repeat ya Wahhab for three or seven nights 100 times after a two cycle midnight prayer with ablution and God'may bless you with your needs.
al-Waḥīd	66	Unique, The	Repeat yā Waḥīd 1000 times when you are alone and in a dark place and you should be freed of fear and delusions.
al-Wajīd	64	Resourceful, The	Repeat yā Wajīd with every morsel of food you eat and you may become light
al-Wakīl	52	Trustee, The	If you are afraid of drowning, being burned in a fire or a similar danger, you should repeat yā Wakīl from time to time to be under God's protection.
al-Walī	55	Friend, The	Recite yā Walī frequently and you are likely to become a Friend of God.

G: List of the Transliteration of the 99 Most Beautiful Names, Their Invocation (dhikr) with an Index to Special Properties

Transliteration	Order	Translation	Invocation
al-Wālī	77	Governor, The	Repeat yā Wālī in your home and it should be free from danger.
al-Wārith	97	Inheritor, The	Recite yā Wārith 100 times at sunrise and you should be free of difficulties. If you recite it often, your work should be fulfilled.
al-Wāsi'	45	Vast, The	Recite yā Wāsi' frequently if you have difficulty earning a living andyou should have good earnings. God may give you contentment and blessings.
al-Ẓāhir	75	Manifest, The	Recite yā Ẓāhir 500 times and the Divine Light may enter your heart.

G: List of the Transliteration of the 99 Most Beautiful Names, Their Invocation (dhikr) with an Index to Special Properties

Need	Name
Anger, God subside your	al-Māni‘
Appeal answered	al-‘Alīm
appeal answered	al-Mutakabbir
Appeal answered	al-Samī‘
Appeal answered	al-Wahhāb
Awareness, develop keen	al-Raḥmān
Bad habit, freed of	al-Khabīr
Blessed	al-Barr
Blessed by God and His people	al-Ra’ūf
Calamities, protected from	al-Ḥafīẓ
Compelled to do something against your wishes, not	al-Jabbār
Composure, maintain	al-Shakūr
Contentment, gain	al-Ghanī
Day of Judgment, ease of	al-Muḥṣī
Desires of attraction to pleasure, conquer	al-Qahhār
Despair, temporary, relief from	al-Ghafūr
Destiny opened	al-‘Alī
Difficulties cleared up	al-Rashīd
Difficulties disappear	al-Badī‘
Difficulties eases	al-Muta‘ālī
Difficulties eased	al-Matīn
Difficulties in work overcome	al-Ḥakīm
Difficulties, facing	al-Qādir
Difficulties, free of	al-Bāqī
Difficulties, free of,	al-Wārith
Difficulties, rescued from	al-‘Afū
Dignity in eyes of others, develop	al-Mu‘izz
Drowning, afraid of	al-Wakīl
Earning a living, difficulty of	al-Wāsi‘
Enemy's harm, free from	al-Khāfiḍ
Enemy's harm, free from	al-Qādir
Enemy, captured by	al-Wahhāb
Enemy, defeat an	al-Qawī
Enemy, destroy your	al- Mumīt
Enemy, freed from harm by	al-Qawī
Enemy, overcome your	al-Qahhār
Enemy, victorious over	al-Muntaqim
Esteem among people	Dhu ’l-Jalāl
Esteem in eyes of others	al-Baṣīr
Esteem in this world, gain	al-Karīm
Esteem, gain	al-Kabīr
Esteem, gain	Mālik al-Mulk
Faith raised	al-‘Alī
Faith, continue to have	al-Mujīb
Family life, good	al-Māni‘
Family, safety of	al-Raqīb
Fear and delusions, free of	al-Wahīd
Fear none but God	al-Mu‘izz
Fear of God, gain	al-Bā‘ith
Fear of harm from a jealous person	al-Mudhill
Fever, relief from	al-Ghafūr
Fire, afraid of	al-Wakīl
Friend of God, become a	al-Walī
Friendliness of others increased	al-Raḥīm
Friends, keep	al-Qayyūm
Glory, gain	al-Majīd
God's sake only, act for	al-Khāliq
God, gain benevolence of	al-Muta‘ālī
God, grow closer to	al-Ḍārr
Good end, have a	al-Akhir
Good life, lead a	al-Akhir
Grave, safe from punishment	al-Qābiḍ
Hardship, not exposed to	al-Jabbār
Harm of idol/ego, free from	al-Mu’min
Harm of idol/ego, free from	al-Muqsiṭ
Harm, avoid	al-Nāfi‘
Harm, preserve something planted from	al-Ḥalīm
Harmed, free of being	al-Ḥasīb
Headache, relief from	al-Ghafūr
Heart expand	al-Quddūs
Heart heavy	al-Shakūr
Heart, enlighten your	al-Mājid
Heart, freed of a heavy	al-Raḥmān
Heart, freed of rust	al-Fattāḥ
Heart, only love of God in your	al-Mu’akhkhir
Heavy burden, weight of a	al-Muḥyīi
Hidden meaning, attain	al-Ṣamad
Hidden meanings, know	al-Ḥakam
Hidden work, know about	al-‘Alīm
Home free of danger	al-Wālī
Honor, attain higher sense of	al-Rāfi‘
Hunger, safe from	al-Qābiḍ
Idol/ego, victory over	al-Fattāḥ
Illuminate heart	al-‘Alīm
Illumination of inner being	al-Muhaymin

G: List of the Transliteration of the 99 Most Beautiful Names, Their Invocation (dhikr) with an Index to Special Properties

NEED	NAME	NEED	NAME
Intuition, receive	al-'Alīm	Sick person	al-Ṣalam
Jealous person, fear of harm from	al-Mudhill	Sick, if you are	al-Ḥayy
Jealousy, free of fear of	al-Ḥasīb	Sickness, freed from	al-Laṭīf
Khidr, meet	al-Razzāq	Sorrows, rescued from	al-'Afū
Life, have a long	al-Ḥayy	Spiritual knowledge, gain	al-Hādī
Light enter your heart	al-Ẓāhir	Spiritual state, attain higher	
Light in your heart, gain	al-Nūr	Sustenance met, have	al-Razzāq
Light, become	al-Wajīd	Traveler return safely	al-Mu'īd
Light, Divine, revealed	al-'Alīm	Troubles, rescued from	al-'Afū
Light, gain inner	al-Nūr	Truth, aware of	al-Muqtadir
Light, receive inner	al-Nūr	Truth, see in things	al-Bāṭin
Livelihood insufficient	al-Wahhāb	Unveiling, receive	al-'Alīm
Lonliness, freed from	al-Laṭīf	Violence, not exposed to	al-Jabbār
Losing something	al-Mubdi'	Work fulfilled	al-Wārith
Lost objects, to find	al-Jāmi'	Work, hard, become easy	al-Muṣawwir
Lost, something, try to find	al-Ḥaqq	Work, hard, becomes easy	al-Bāri'
Loved and praised, be	al-Ḥamīd	Wrongdoings forgiven	al-Ghaffār
Manners, developing good	al-Muqīt	Wronged by another, freed from being	al-Qahhār
Memory, develop good	al-Raḥmān	Wronged, free of fear of	al-Ḥasīb
Merit, attain higher sense of	al-Rāfi'		
Misfortune, free from	al-Barr		
Need of others, freed from	al-Bāsiṭ		
Need, free of	al-'Azīz		
Needs fulfilled	al-Awwal		
Oppressor, never fall into the grip of	al-Ṣamad		
Oppressor, safe from an	al-Mudhill		
Passions, control	al-Mumīt		
Peace, gain inner	al-Qahhār		
People obey you	al-'Adl		
Poverty, freed from	al-Laṭīf		
Poverty, not suffer	al-Razzāq		
Property, safety of	al-Raqīb		
Purpose, attain your	al-Muqsiṭ		
Quarrel among two people	al-Wadūd		
Rebellious child become obedient	al-Shahīd		
Repentance accepted	al-Tawwāb		
Respect, gain	al-Kabīr		
Respected by others	al-Malik		
Revered among people	al-Jalīl		
Richness, attain higher sense	al-Rāfi'		
Robed, free of fear of being	al-Ḥasīb		
Self, safety of	al-Raqīb		
Self-sufficient, become	al-Mughnī		
Severity, not exposed to	al-Jabbār		

Notes

Preface

1. See *God's Will Be Done*, Volume II: *Moral Healer's Handbook: The Psychology of Spiritual Chivalry.*

2. It should be noted that God is beyond gender but uses the pronoun He in the Quran because in the Arabic langauge, the masculine pronoun is used when reference is to the masculine third person singular or the masculine and feminine third person singular.

3. The word *wajh* (Face or Presence) is used most frequently in the Quran with the meaning of the human self (*nafs, dhat*) (see 2:112, 3:20, 4:12r, 6:79, 10:105, 30:30, 30:43, 31:22, 39:24). When used in regard to God, it refers to how people act out of a desire for the Presence of Face of God (2:272, 13:22, 92:20); desire to make for the Presence of God (6:52, 18:27, 30:38, 39); act for the sake of the Presence of God (76:9). Then, "*To God belongs the East and the West; wherever you turn, there is the Presence of God*" (2:115); "*Everything perishes except His Presence,*" (28:88); "*Whoever is upon (the earth) perishes yet the Presence of the Lord abides, He of Majssty and Generosity*" (55:27).

Overview

1. Naraqī, p. 45.

2. Ṭūsī, p. 39

3. *Nicomachaen Ethics,* 2.9.1109b24-28, quoted by Algazel, *Iḥyā.*

4. See *God's Will Be Done*, Volume II: *Moral Healer's Handbook: The Psychology of Spiritual Chivalry.*

5. Arabic is considered to be a sacred langauge by Muslims because God chose that langauge in which to disclose Self.

6. Algazel, *Iḥyā*, pp. 106-110.

7. The Muslim day of rest and day of the obligatory congregational prescribed prayer.

8. Muslim, *Musāfirīn*, p. 168.

9. Tirmidhi, Du'a, p. 44; Ibn Mājā, *Ṣiyam*, p. 34.

10. Muslim, Salāt, p. 215.

11. Muslim, Salāt, p. 212.

12. Abū Dāwūd, Witr, p. 23.

13. Algazel, *Iḥyā*, p. 347.

14. Tirmidhī, Da'awāt, p. 76.

15. Bukhārī, Tawḥid, p. 31.

16. Muslim, Dhikr, p. 9.

17. Tirmidhī, Da'awāt, p. 65.

18. Muslim, Jihād, p. 107.

19. Bukhārī, Da'awāt, p. 22.

20. Ibn Ḥanbal, *Musnad*, IV. 54.

21. Naqshbandi Dihlavi, *Jawāhir al-khamseh*, p. 212.

22. Ibn Khaldun, *Muqaddimah*, pp. 171-181.

23. Quoted by R. Guenon, *Symbolism of the Cross* p. 68.

24. al-Būnī, *Shams*, p. 78.

25. See *God's Will Be Done*, Volume II: *Moral Healer's Handbook: The Psychology of Spiritual Chivalry.*

26. Ibn Khaldun, *op. cit.*

27. Ibn Khaldun, *op. cit.*

Part II: The Process of Moral Healing for Spiritual Warriors Through Psychoethics

Chapter One: Moral Healing of the Attraction to Pleasure Function of the Self Through Acquiring Temperance

1. Algazel, *Iḥyā*, III. 1493, 1496, 1507.
2. *Ibid.*, IV. 3.2316.
3. *Ibid.*, IV. 3.2317.
4. *Ibid.*, IV. 3.2317.
5. *Ibid.*, IV. 3.2319.
6. Rūmī, *Mathnawī.*
7. Kāshānī. *Misbah al-hidāya.*
8. Abū Naṣr Ṣarraj, *Kitāb al-luma'.*
9. Anṣārī, *Ṭabaqāt*, p. 561.
10. Algazel, *Mizān*,, p. 98.
11. Tūsī, *Akhlāq*, p. 83.
12. *Ibid.*, p. 83.
13. Rūmī, *Mathnawī.*
14. Algazel, *Iḥyā*, IV. 4.2423-24.
15. *Ibid.*, IV. 4.2464.

Chapter Two: Moral Healing of the Avoidance of Harm/Pain Function of the Self Through Acquiring Courage

1. Hanbal, *Musnad* in Muslim, pp. 242, 258.
2. *Sahih Muslim.*
3. *Sahih Bukhārī*, Book IV, p. 179.
4. *Sahih Muslim.*
5. Rūmī, *Mathnawī.*
6. Muhāsibī, *Muḥāsabal.* p. 45.
7. Kāshānī, *Misbah al-hidayah*, p. 394.
8. *Sahih Bukhari*, Vol. 4, p. 179; Vol. 9, p. 141.
9. Algazel, *Ihyā*, p. 252.
10. Aṭṭār, *Tadhkirat al-awliyā'*, p. 503.
11. *Ibid.*, p. 280.
12. Based on Sign 25:63 of the Quran.
13. See Javad Nurbakhsh, *Sufism V*, p. 101.
14. Aṭṭār, *Tadhkirat al-awliyā'*, p. 492.
15. 'Alī ibn Abī Ṭālib, *Nahj al-balaghah*, p. 117.
16. Anṣārī, *Ṭabaqāt aṣ-ṣufiya*, p. 233.
17. Abū Naṣr Sarrāj, *Al-luma'.*
18. Junayd, *Fi'l farq bain al-ikhlāṣ.*
19. Algazel, *Iḥyā*, III. 6, 1979.

Chapter Three: Moral Healing of the Cognitive Function of Self Through Acquiring Wisdom

1. Algazel, *Mizān*, p. 84.
2. Sherif, p. 42.
3. Naraqī, p. 64.
4. Algazel, *Mizān.*, pp. 84-85.
5. Avicennā, *Shifā'*, Metaphysics, II, 455.
6. Nurbakhsh, *Sufism V*, p. 79.
7. Anṣārī, *Manazil al-sa'irin*, p. 136.
8. Shāh Ni'matullāhī Wālī. *Risalāhā.*
9. Anṣārī, *Ṣad maydān*, p. 45.
10. Munawwir, *Aṣrār al-tawḥid*, p. 292.

11. Aṭṭār, *Ilāhīnama*, p. 53.
12. Sulamī, Abu 'Abd Raḥmān. *Ṭabaqāt aṣ-ṣufiya*, p. 321.
13. Aṭṭār, *Tadhkirat al-awliyā*", p. 149.
14. *Ibid.*, p. 753.
15. Anṣārī, *Ṭabaqāt aṣ-ṣufiya*, p. 515.
16. Aṭṭār, *Tadhkirat al-awliyā'*, p. 757.
17. Algazel, *Kimīyā as-sadat*, pp. 13-16.
18. Aṭṭār, *Tadhkirat al-awliyā'*, p. 745.
19. Junayd, *Risala*, pp. 47-51.
20. Qushari, *Al-risālat al-Qushariya*, p. 296.
21. Anonymous author, *Khulāsā-yī sharḥ-i ta'aruf.* p. 312.
22. *Ibid.*
23. See Javad Nurbakhsh, *Sufism IV.*
24. Algazel, *Maqasid*, p. 110.
25. Jamī, *Lawa'ih.*
26. Anṣārī, *Ṣad maydan*, pp. 326-327.
27. *Ibid.*, pp. 322-323.
28. Jurjānī, Mir Sayyed Sharif. *Al-ta'rifat.*
29. Sulamī, *Ṭabiqāt aṣ-ṣufiya*, p. 47.
30. Qushari, *Risalā*, pp. 446.
31. Aṭṭār, *Tadhkirat al-awliyā'*, p. 710.
32. See Javad Nurbakhsh, *Sufism IV.*
33. Sherif, p. 103.
34. Algazel, *Iḥyā*, IV. 9. 2803.
35. *Ibid.*, IV. 9. 2822-44.
36. Sherif, p. 106.

Chapter Four: Centering the Self with Justice

1. Naraqī, p. 36.

Bibliography

Abū Dāwūd. *al-Sunan.* Cairo, 1950-51.

Abū Naṣr Ṣarraj. *Kitāb al-lumā'*. Ed. R. A. Nicholson. London, 1914.

(Algazel). Ghazālī, Muḥammad Aḥmad. *al-Mizān al-Amal.* Cairo: Matba'at Khurdistan al-Ilmiyyah.

(Algazel). Ghazālī, Muḥammad Aḥmad. *Ihya ulum al-din.* Trans. Fazul Karim. Dehli: Taj Company, 1968.

(Algazel). *Kimīyā-yi ṣadat.* Cairo, 1963.

'Alī ibn Abī Ṭālib. *Nahj al-balāghah.* Cairo, 1972.

Anonymous author, *Khulāṣā-yi sharḥ-i-ta'aruf.* Tehran, 1982.

Anṣārī, Khwāja 'Abdullāh. *Manāzil al-sā'irin.* Ed. S. Laugier de Beaurecueil. Cairo, 1962.

Anṣārī, Khwāja 'Abdullāh, *Ṣad Maydān.* Ed. Rawān Farhādī. Kabul, 1976.

Anṣārī, Khwāja 'Abdullāh. *Ṭabaqāt aṣ-ṣufiya.* Ed. A. Habibi, Kabul, 1347/1968.

Ardalan, Nader and Laleh Bakhtiar. *The Sense of Unity: The Sufi Tradition in Persian Architecture.* Chicago: University of Chicago Press, 1973.

Aṭṭār, Farīd ul-Din. *Illāhīnamā.* Ed. Helmut Ritter, Tehran, 1980.

Aṭṭār, Farīd ul-Din, *Tadhkirat al-awliyā'*. Ed. Muḥammad Esti'lāmī. Tehran, 1975.

Avicenna, *Shifā'*. Cairo, 1982.

Bakhtiar, Laleh. *God's Will Be Done: Moral Healer's Handbook: The Psychology of Spiritual Chivalry.* Chicago: The Institute of Traditional Psychoethics and Guidance, 1994, Vol. II.

Bakhtiar, Laleh. *God's Will Be Done: Traditional Psychoethics and PersonalityParadigm.* Chivalry. Chicago: The Institute of Traditional Psychoethics and Guidance, 1994. Vol. I.

Bakhtiar, Laleh. *SUFI Expressions of the Mystic Quest.* London: Thames and Hudson, 1976.

Bukhārī, 'Abdullāh. *Sharḥ al-ta'arruf.* Ed. A. Rajā'i. Tehran. 1970.

Bukhari, Muhammad. *al-Jāmi' al-Saḥiḥ.* Ed. M. Ludolf Krehl and Theodor W. Juynboll. Leiden, 1862-1908.

Būnī, al-. *Shams al-ma'ārif al-kubrā.* Cairo: nd. 1:78.

Guenon, Rene. *Symbolism of the Cross.* Trans. A. Macnab. London: Luzac, 1975.

Ibn Hanbal, Ahmad. *al-Musnad.* Cairo, 1954-6.
Ibn Khaldun. *Muqaddimah.* Cairo, 1904.
Ibn Mājā. *al-Sunan.* Ed. Muḥammad Fu'ād 'Abd al-Bāqī. Cairo, 1952-54.
Junayd, Abu'l Qasim. In A. H. Abdul Qādir, *The Life, Personality and Writings of al-Junayd.* London, 1962.
Jurjani, 'Alī ibn Muḥammad. *Al-tarifat.* Ed. G. Flugel. Leipsig, 1945.
Kashani, Miṣbāh al-hidāya. Ed. Muḥammad Kamāl Ibrāhīm. Egypt, 1984.
Kashani, 'Abd al-Razzāq. *Tuḥfat al-ikhwān fikhaṣa'iṣ al-fityān.* In *Rasa'il-i jawān mardān.* Ed. M. Ṣarrāf. Tehran: Institut Franco-Iranien, 1973.
Miskawayh, Ibn. *Tahdhīb al-akhlāq.* Trans. Constantine Zurayk. Beirut: American University of Beirut, 1968.
Muhasibi, Ḥārith b. Asad. *Muḥāsabal al-nufūs.* MS, Cairo, Tas. Sh. 3.
Munawwir, Muḥammad. *Asrār al-tawḥīd.* Ed. Dhabiullāh Ṣafā. Tehran, 1928.
Muslim, b. al-Hajjaj. *Saḥīḥ.* Cairo, 1334.
Naqshbandi Dihlavi, Maulanā Mirzā Muḥammad. *Jawahir al-khamseh..* Lahore, Pakistan: Maktabah Raḥmāniyah.
Naraqi, Muḥammad Mahdi ibn Abi Dharr. *Jāmī al-ṣa'dat.* Tehran: Ilm Press, 1987.
Nurbakhsh, Javad. *Sufism.* London: Khanaghah Nimatullahi. 5 vols.
Qushārī, Abu'l Qāṣim. *Al-risālat al-Qushairiyā.* Ed. by A. Mahmud. Cairo, 1972-74.
Rumi, Jalāl al-Din. *Mathnawī.* Ed. R. A. Nicholson, Tehran, 1977. 6 vols.
Shah Nimatullahi Wali, *Risālahā.* Ed. Javad Nurbakhsh. Tehran, 1978. 4 vols.
Sherif, M. A. *Ghazali's Theory of Virtue.* New York: SUNY, 1975.
Sulami, Abu 'Abd Rahman. *Ṭabaqāt al-ṣufiyā.* Eds. Johannes Peterson. Leiden. 1960.
Tirmidhi, al-. *al-Sunan.* Medina, 1384-7/1964-7.
Ṭūsī, Naṣir al-Din. *Akhlāq al-Nasirī.* Trans. G. Wickens, London: George Allen and Unwin, 1964.

Index

A

abādī 61
abaser 72, 138
Abaser, The 18
abasing 74
'Abdullāh 225
abīd 129
able 107
Able, The 29, 47, 48, 153, 214
Abraham 22, 161
abscess 180
Absolute 7, 115
abstinence 149
Abu Musa 225
abuse 88
Acceptor of Repentance, The 52
Acts 106
Adam 67, 84, 145, 166, 200, 203
'*adl* 102, 144, 231
'Adl, al- 21, 103, 145, 214
affect 111
'*afu* 91, 193, 233
'Afū, al- 53, 54, 92, 204
aḥad 106, 183, 190, 232
Aḥad, al- 46, 106
akhir 193, 232
Akhir, al 108, 199
Algazel 13, 14, 67, 68, 72, 73, 77, 78, 84, 90, 92, 94, 95, 109, 124, 193
'*alī* 103, 154, 179, 231
'Alī, al- 26, 155
alim 101, 131, 166
'Alīm, al- 17, 24, 29, 31, 34, 39, 42, 103, 135, 230
alive 183
All-Hearing, The 101, 103, 142, 144
All-Knowing, The 144
All-Seeing, The 101, 103, 144
Allāh 7
Allāh al-'Alīm 17
Allāhū akbar 13
Altruism 69
altruism 77, 78
ambition 48, 197
Amīin, al- 174
amintū billāhī 201
amr bil ma'ruf 12, 120, 138
Angel of Death 143
angel of death 155
anger 79, 80, 82, 83, 133, 137
anger, inappropriate 80, 81, 86, 99, 115, 122, 141
angur 123
animal self 186
animal skin 147
Anṣārī 99, 190
ant (s) 19, 134, 159
anthropomorphism 20
apple 218
appraiser 74, 75
Appraiser, The 42
Arab (s) 123, 216
Arab horses 216
Arabic grammar 158
arbiter 102, 138
Arbiter, The 20, 103, 144
architect 145
arrogant 140
aṣ-ṣalām alaykūm 10
Aspiration 96, 99
aspiration 100
astaphil 123
atonement 92
Aṭṭār 99, 103, 191
attraction to pleasure 69, 71, 75, 78, 80, 96, 124
Attributes 106
Attributes and Acts 93
avenger 91
Avenger, The 53, 54
Avicenna 96

avoidance of harm 71, 79, 83, 93, 96, 111, 124
aware 103, 138
Aware, The 23, 39, 146
awwal 193, 232
Awwal, al- 108, 199
aẓalī 61
'*aẓīm* 103, 150, 151
'Aẓīm, al- 24, 30, 31
'azīz 12, 100, 115, 128, 229, 231
'Azīz, al- 11, 153
Azrael 155, 156

B

badī' 109, 217, 233
Badī', al- 60, 223
Badr 36
Baghdad 152
bā'ith 74, 75
Ba'ith, al- 35, 165
balance 115
Baluchistan 150
baqā 9
bāqī 61, 109, 217, 233
Bāqī, al- 61, 223
barber 151
bāri' 131, 132
Bāri', al- 13, 72, 131, 229
barley 215
barr 193, 233
Barr, al- 52, 109, 202
Baṣīr, al- 101, 103, 144
bāsiṭ 72, 138, 230
Bāsiṭ, al- 17, 181
bāṭin 193, 233
Bāṭin, al- 50, 108, 199
Battle of Uhud 164
bear 128
beatuy 14
Beautiful, The 30
beauty 30
bedouin 160
bee (s) 60, 181
beginner 75
Beginner, The 42, 43
beginning 181
behavior 111
being alive 184
believer (s) 9, 83, 84
beneficial 78
Bestower, The 15, 35, 86, 133, 165
Bilqis 167, 168, 169
bird 140, 189
Bistāmī 203
boasting 80
boatman 158
Bountiful, The 213
building 146

C

Caliph 'Alī 208, 215
caliph 154
Calph 'Umar 210
calumny 88
camel (s) 184, 202, 203, 210
cat 147, 189
chastity 185
Chinese artists 194
cleansed 229
clement 93
Clement, The 54, 207
clot of blood 37
cloud 220
cognition 111
cognitive faculty 95
command to the positive 138
commanding to the positive 84
commands 12
community 131
Companions 142
Compassion 80
compassion 83, 84, 153
compassionate 85, 115, 121, 228
Compassionate, The 8, 9, 83, 207

Compeller, The 7, 8, 12, 71, 128
Concealer of Faults, The 25, 54, 86, 92
concealer of faults 152
conscience 71
Consciousness 96
consciousness 93, 95, 146
consciousness of God 115
Constancy 97
constancy 106
constrictor 72, 138, 230
Constrictor, The 17, 181
Constrictor-Expander 18
Contentment 97
contentment 105
couage 115
counsel themselvese 144
counsel to the positive 120, 140
Counseling to the Positive 116, 137
counseling the self 145
counseling to the positive 12, 84
courage 79, 80
Courtesy 80
courtesy 85
courtier (s) 123, 208
covenant 103
cowardice 82
creation 115, 228
creations, new 38
Creative Process, Entering the 116
creativity 136
Creator 12, 14, 89, 92, 95, 167
Creator of the Beneficial, The 58, 215
Creator, The 13, 72, 131
creatures 9
criminal 146

D

ḍārr 78, 207, 215, 233
Ḍārr, al- 58
Day of Judgment 34, 132, 198, 207, 211
Day of Resurrection 38
deaf 143
deceit 88
desire 137
desire for evil 127
desires, inappropriate 99
detachment 105
Dhū'l Jalāl 55, 109, 209
dhū' l jalāl 207
dishonorer 72, 74, 138
Dishonorer, The 18
dispute 89
Divine Presence 74
Divine Attributes 198
Divine Decree 21, 184
Divine Grace 44
Divine Law 223
Divine Light 83
Divine Origin 91
Divine Tradition 83, 115, 144
Divine Unity 223
Divine wrath 102
dog 160
dragon 176, 184

E

earth 12
ego 184
elephants 134
emotion 95
enricher 93
Enricher, The 57, 214
envy 127, 180
equitable 77
Equitable, The 55, 211
Essence 38, 55, 106
eternal 99
eternal life 16
Eternal, The 46, 47, 61, 106
everlasting 109, 217
Everlasting, The 61, 223

evil, Absolute 10
Exalted, The 52, 109
exalter 72
Exalter, The 18
exalting 74
expander 72, 138, 230
Expander, The 17, 181

F

Face 7
faith 115, 152
Faith, The Giver of 229
false self 100, 183
falsehood 140
falsity 230
fame 80
fattāḥ 86, 131, 134
Fattāḥ, al- 16. 86, 135, 230
faults 150
fear 72
fear of anything other than God 82
fikr 108
Finder, The 213
firm 105
Firm, The 40, 41
firmness 41
First, The 108, 199
fish 145
fitraṭ Allāh 76, 137
flawless 100, 115, 124
Flawless, The 10, 127
forbearance 149
forebearer 149
Forebearer, The 24, 86
forgetfulness 48
Forgiver 131
forgiver 84, 132, 153
Forgiver, The 14, 25, 54, 92, 131
fowl 145
fox 162
fraud 127
free will 9, 71
Friend, The 41, 90, 175
friends of God 172
futuwwah 150

G

Gabriel 164
gatherer 77
Gatherer, The 56, 212
Generosity 81
generous 87, 159
Generous, The 31, 35, 160, 161, 163, 165, 211
gentle 138, 145
ghaffār 84, 132, 153, 229
Ghaffār, al- 14, 25, 92, 131
ghafūr 150, 152, 231
Ghafūr, al- 25, 86, 92
ghanī 109, 207, 233
Ghanī, al- 57, 213
ghayrat 84
Giver of Faith, The 11, 127, 229
glass 219
Glorious, The 35, 165
Glory 55
glory 13, 188
gnat 145, 166, 175
gnosis 230
God is Greater 13
God knows best 17
God Wills 106
God's Command 129, 156
God's Will 12, 63, 71, 86, 87, 94, 100, 129, 130, 194, 195, 208, 233
gold 171
good deeds 104
Goodness, Source of All 52
gossip 88
governor 95, 200
grape 123
great 155
Great, The 27, 29
greatness, inner 103

greed 180
Greek 123
Greek artists 194
guardian 83, 84, 128
Guardian, The 11, 85
Guarding against 127
Guide and Teacher, Serving as 118
guide 217, 221
Guide, The 60
guide, inner 93
Gulshan-i-rāz 166

H

hādī 93, 217, 221, 233
Hādī, al- 60
ḥadith 58, 132, 160
ḥadith qudsī 115, 197
ḥafīẓ 74, 150, 155, 157, 231
Ḥafīẓ, al- 27, 31, 58, 156, 214
ḥakam 102, 138, 144, 231
Ḥakam, al- 20, 103, 144
ḥakīm 103, 159, 163, 232
Ḥakīm, The 33
ḥalīm 149, 150, 171, 231
Ḥalīm, al- 24, 86
hamdullāh, al- 179
ḥamīd 172, 179, 232
Ḥamīd, al- 41, 42, 105, 179
Hamzah 85
Hannah 195
ḥaqq 39, 104
Ḥaqq, al- 39, 167, 232
harmful 78
ḥasīb 87, 150, 158, 231
Ḥasīb, al- 29
hatred 127, 180
ḥayy 105, 183, 232
Ḥayy, al- 43
He is the Everlasting 62
heart 115, 122
heavens 164
Hereafter 224
Hidden, The 50, 51, 108, 199
ḥifẓ 58
high-mindedness 87
highest 179
Highest, The 26, 27, 155
holy 99
Holy, The 10, 99
honor 141, 230
honorer 72, 74, 138
Honorer, The 18
hope 72, 73
Hope-Fear 69
horse 7
humanity 115
Humility 80
humility 84, 85
hunger 126
huntsman 160
huwā 'l Baqī 62
hypocrisy 96, 153, 157

I

Iblis 203
Ibn Miskāwayh 96
Ibrāhīm ibn Adham 209
iḥṣān 149
imagination 218
imaginative function 217
importance 11
inab 123
inaccessibility 11, 13
inaccessibility 13
incomparable 12, 100, 128
Incomparable, The 11
India 123, 156
ingratitude 88, 89
Inheritor, The 62, 78
ink 33
inner guide 93
Instinctive Motivation, Perfecting 118
intellect, the 88, 217, 218

intention 71, 104
intrepidity 87
intuition 217, 219
ithār 77, 78, 227

J

jabbār 115
Jabbār, al- 12, 71, 128, 129
jackal 146, 178
jalīl 103, 159, 193, 231
Jalīl, al- 29, 30, 35, 159, 163, 165
jāmi‘ 77, 211, 233
Jāmi‘, al- 56, 212
Jamīl, al- 30
javanmardī 150
Jesus 15, 178, 204
Jesus, Prophet 10
jihād 185
jinn 145, 210
just 102, 144
Just, The 21, 22, 103, 145, 214
justice 22, 39, 85, 95, 111, 112, 144, 200

K

Kabah 213
kabīr 103, 155
Kabīr, al- 27, 29
karīm 87, 159, 232
Karīm, al- 31, 35, 160, 161, 163, 165
Kāshāni 74
khabīr 103, 138, 166
Khabīr, al- 23, 39, 146
khāfiḍ 72, 74, 138, 140, 230
Khāfiḍ, al- 18
khāliq 131
Khāliq, al- 13, 72, 131, 172
Khidr 139
kindness 149
King of Absolute Sovereignty 54
king 122, 208
knower 101
Knower, The 17, 24, 29, 31, 34, 39, 103, 135, 136

L

lamp 218
Last, The 50, 108, 199
laṭīf 102, 138, 145, 231
Laṭīf, al- 15, 23, 103, 146
Law 68, 88, 91, 133, 197, 207
liberating the self 149
life-giver 76
Life-Giver, The 43
light 217
Light, The 59
lion (s) 134, 150, 162
Living, The 43, 44, 105
Lord of Majesty and Generosity 55, 109, 209
love of wealth 80
loving 164
Loving, The 34, 35, 89, 153
lump of flesh 37
Luqmān 133
lust, inappropriate 122

M

magnificent 103
Magnificent, The 24, 30, 31, 153
maintainer 150, 157
Maintainer, The 28, 29, 87
Majestic The 29, 30, 35, 159, 160, 163, 165
Majesty 13, 55
mājid (*majīd*) 104, 105, 159, 183, 188, 232
Mājid, al- (Majīd, al-) 35, 45, 165
Maker of Perfect Harmony, The 13, 14, 72, 131
Makkah 174
makramā 55
Mālik al-Mulk 54
malik 95, 99, 100, 115, 121, 122,

124, 141, 228
mālik al-mulk 77, 207, 233
Malik, al- 9, 54
māni' 58, 78, 207, 214
Māni', al- 58, 215
Manifest, The 50, 51, 108, 199
ma' rifah 60
marriage 68
Mary 195
matīn 105, 172, 232
Matīn, al 40
merchant 151
Merciful 9, 22
merciful 115, 121
Merciful, The 8, 83, 211, 214
mercilessness 180
mercy 8, 73, 115, 120, 121, 146
Messenger (s) 8, 9, 36, 37, 58, 84, 93, 102, 108, 121, 131, 142, 155, 160, 163, 164, 184, 185, 201, 210, 211, 214, 221, 225
minister 157
Moderation 69
moderation 68, 72, 75, 76, 79, 101, 115, 149, 171
Moral Reasonableness 81, 149
Moral Reasonableness, Developing the 116
moral goodness 85
moral healing 68
moral reasonableness 158, 159
moral-seeker 67
morally reasonable person 150, 153
Moses 135, 136, 139
mosque 222
mosquito 175
Most Beautiful Names 7, 69, 73, 80, 81, 111, 115, 132, 153, 201, 212
Most Beautiful Signs of God 115
Mt. Tur 202
mu' adhdhin 125
mu' akhkhir 76, 193
Mu'akhkhir, al- 48, 197, 232
mubdi' 75, 172, 181
Mubdi', al- 42, 181, 232
mudhill 72, 74, 138, 141, 230
Mudhill, al- 18
mughnī 93, 207, 233
Mughni, al- 57, 213, 214
Muḥammad 13, 139, 221
muhaymin 83, 84, 115, 127, 128
Muhaymin, al- 11, 85
muḥṣī 74, 75, 172, 179, 232
Muḥṣī, al- 57, 179
muḥyī 76, 183, 184
Muḥyī, al- 43
mu'īd 43, 75, 172, 181
Mu'īd, al- 42, 181
mu'izz 72, 74, 138, 141, 230
Mu'izz, al- 18
mujīb 163, 232
Mujīb, al- 32, 89
mule 202
mulitplicity in unity 190
Mulk, al- 54
multiplicity 190
multitheism 96
mumin 83, 84, 115
Mu'min, al- 11, 127, 229
mumīt 76, 183, 184, 232
Mumīt, al- 43
muntaqim 91, 203, 233
Muntaqim, al- 53, 203
muqaddim 76, 193
Muqaddim, al- 48, 197, 232
muqīt 150, 157, 231
Muqīt, al- 28, 87
muqsiṭ 77, 207, 210, 233
Muqsiṭ, al- 55, 211
muqtadir 76, 193, 232
Muqtadir, al- 47
murawwah 85, 150
muṣawwir 131, 132
Musawwir, al- 13, 72, 131, 229

musk-pod 192
Muslim 142
muta'ālī 193, 233
Muta'ālī, al- 109, 201
mutakabbir 100, 115, 223
Mutakabbir, al- 31, 100, 130
mystic 121, 123
mysticism 230
mystics 50

N

nāfi' 78, 207, 233
Nāfi', al- 58, 215
nafs 9, 100
nahy an al-munkar 12, 120, 138
Names 7
Names and Qualities 80
Names of God 7
Naraqi 95
negative 145, 172
Negative, Trying to Prevent the Development of 116, 137
negative, development of 138
nightingales 83
Nimrod 175
Ninety-Nine Most Beautiful Names 80, 227
Ninety-Nine Names 115
Noble Character Development 117, 118
Noble, The 35, 45
nūr 217, 233
Nūr, al- 59

O

objectivity 154
one 106
One, The 46, 106
oneness 190
opener 86, 134
Opener, The 16, 86
oppression 145
oppressor 89
originator 109
Originator, The 60, 61, 181, 182, 223
others 191
overconsciousness 96

P

Paradise 176, 211
pardoner 91
Pardoner, The 53, 54, 92, 204
parrot (s) 151, 152
passions 79, 89, 149
Patience 81
patience 48, 93, 94, 140, 149, 226
patient 93, 111
Patient, The 7, 64, 223, 225
peace 10
peacock 146, 185
pen 159
perfect harmony 131, 132
Perfecting their Instinctive Perception 117
perfection 14
perseverance 48, 87
Persian 123
Personality 55
Piety 69, 74, 75, 201
Plato 111
pomegranate 219
pork 68
positive disposition 73, 75, 93
positive resolve 71
positive, prevent the development of 141
postponer 76
Postponer, The 48
powerful 76
Powerful, The 47, 48
Praised, The 41
praiseworthy 172, 203
praiseworthy actions 72

Praiseworthy, The 105, 179
prayer 125, 152, 195
preconsciousness 96
predestination 21
prescribed prayer 152
Presence 7, 55
preserver 74, 150
Preserver, The 27, 28, 31, 58, 156, 214
preserving 58
prevent the development of the negative 12, 120, 140
preventing the negative 85
pride 80, 180
prince 121
probhibitions 12
promoter 76
Promoter, The 48, 197
Prophet 176
prophethood 37, 38
Prophets 17, 48
protection 58
protector 78, 155, 157
Protector, The 58, 156
proud 100
Proud, The 31, 100
provider 133
Provider, The 16, 86
psychoethics 91, 227
punisher 215
Punisher, The 58

Q

qābiḍ 72, 138, 230
Qābiḍ, al- 17, 181
qadar 21
qadar wa qada' 21
qadīm 61
qādir 107, 193, 232
Qādir, al- 29, 42, 47, 153, 214
qahhār 100, 131, 132
Qahhār, al- 15
qawī 105, 172, 232
Qawī, al- 40
qayyūm 105, 183, 186, 232
Qayyūm, al- 44, 186
qiblah 190
quddūs 99, 100, 115, 122, 229
Quddūs, al- 10, 99
Queen of Sheba 167
qunice 218
Quran 1:1 8
Quran 2:28 43
Quran 2:29 17
Quran 2:32 33
Quran 2:37 53
Quran 2:105 24
Quran 2:107 9, 41
Quran 2:112 55
Quran 2:115 32
Quran 2:117 60
Quran 2:235 21
Quran 2:245 17
Quran 2:255 43, 44
Quran 2:257 41
Quran 2:269 163
Quran 3:8 15
Quran 3:9 56
Quran 3:18 56
Quran 3:26 18, 54
Quran 3:35 19
Quran 3:128 204
Quran 3:169 36
Quran 3:173 40
Quran 3:191 16
Quran 4:1 31
Quran 4:6 29
Quran 4:32 174
Quran 4:58 20
Quran 4:85 28
Quran 4:135 85
Quran 5:27 201
Quran 5:119 105
Quran 6:37 47

Quran 6:62 20
Quran 6:73 39
Quran 6:75 22
Quran 6:91 77
Quran 6:101 61
Quran 6:103 23
Quran 7:139 187
Quran 7:156 8
Quran 7:176 124
Quran 8:17 209
Quran 8:46 63
Quran 9:20 124
Quran 9:28 57
Quran 9:112 85
Quran 11:61 32
Quran 11:66 40
Quran 11:87 63
Quran 11:90 34
Quran 13:9 27, 52
Quran 13:11 131
Quran 13:28 90
Quran 15:21 179
Quran 15:23 62
Quran 16:74 7
Quran 16:77 21
Quran 16:92 22
Quran 16:127 94
Quran 17:45 179
Quran 17:70 55
Quran 17:85 37
Quran 17:99 47
Quran 18:45 47
Quran 20:50 60
Quran 20:114 9, 201
Quran 21:101 49
Quran 22:6 39
Quran 22:7 35
Quran 22:60 53
Quran 22:64 42
Quran 23:14 37
Quran 23:96 204
Quran 23:116 31
Quran 24:35 59, 196, 217
Quran 24:40 220
Quran 24:40 221
Quran 25:31 60
Quran 25:43 124
Quran 32:13 49
Quran 32:22 53
Quran 33:21 155
Quran 33:8 105
Quran 33:43 9, 121
Quran 34:13 89
Quran 34:21 27
Quran 34:26 16
Quran 35:14 23
Quran 35:30 25
Quran 38:46 108
Quran 38:82-83 108
Quran 40:16 15, 62
Quran 40:42 15
Quran 41:12 21
Quran 41:46 177
Quran 41:53 22
Quran 42:9 51
Quran 43:4 76
Quran 47:11 41
Quran 47:38 57, 77
Quran 48:1 17
Quran 48:18 77
Quran 50:28 48
Quran 51:58 40
Quran 52:28 52
Quran 53:17 99
Quran 53:39-40 20
Quran 54:11 23
Quran 55:27 55
Quran 56:1-3 18
Quran 56:61 37
Quran 57:3 49, 50
Quran 57:14 19
Quran 57:16 85
Quran 58:6 42

Quran 58:21 41
Quran 59:18 101
Quran 59:23 10, 11, 12, 13
Quran 59:24 13
Quran 60:1 186
Quran 62:1 10
Quran 64:17 24
Quran 65:3 172
Quran 67:3 22
Quran 68:4 175
Quran 69:24 26
Quran 70:23 196
Quran 71:14 37
Quran 79:40 124
Quran 82:6-7 160
Quran 82:13-14 21, 42
Quran 85:15 45
Quran 87:1 26
Quran 87:3 60
Quran 89:27 19
Quran 89:27-28 90
Quran 89:27-30 141
Quran 89:40-41 186
Quran 93:10 163
Quran 99:7-8 177
Quran 100:10 35
Quran 112:2 46
Quran 137, 157, 185, 215

R

rāfi' 72, 74, 138, 140, 141, 230
Rāfi', al- 18
rahamā 8, 115, 121
raḥīm 85, 115, 121, 153, 228
Raḥīm, al- 8, 207
raḥmān 115, 121, 228
Raḥmān, al- 8, 214
raqīb 89, 159, 161, 232
Raqīb, al- 31
rashīd 217, 233
Rashid, al- 63, 78, 223
rational 95
ra' ūf 93, 207, 233
Ra'ūf, al- 54, 207
razzāq 131, 133
Razzāq, al- 16, 86, 230
reason 71, 79, 82, 115, 217
rebellion 84
rebelliousness 74
recklessness 82
reckoner 87, 150, 179
Reckoner, The 29, 179
Religiously Cultured Person 116
rememberer 111
Remembrance 97, 108
remembrance of God 88
Repentance 81
repentance 91, 92
Repentance, The Acceptor of 52
repenter 91, 92, 202
Repenter, The 202
Resolve 69
resolve 71
resourceful 105
Resourceful, The 45
Responder to Prayer, The 32, 89
restorer 75
Restorer, The 42, 43, 181
restsorer 181
resurrection 10, 37, 38, 48
resurrector 74, 75
Resurrector, The 35, 36, 38, 165
retribution 31
revenge 203
Rewarder of Thankfulness, The 25, 87, 153
Rich, The 57, 213
Right in Guidance, The 63, 78, 223
right 150
Rightly-Guided 207
Rightly-Guided Caliph 154
rose 83
ruler 100
Rumi 83, 115, 129, 134, 138, 139,

142, 185, 191, 212, 223

S

Saba 167
ṣabur 93, 217, 233
Ṣabur, al- 63, 223, 225
Safety 11
salām 100, 115, 124
Salām, al- 10, 127
ṣalāt 152
salvation 10
ṣamad 99, 183, 191, 232
Ṣamad, al- 46, 106
samī' 231
Samī', al- 101, 103, 142
Satan 81, 84, 138
satanic temptations 132
scab 180
scholar 158
scorpion 177
security 11
seeking of pleasures 48
Self 55, 115
self-centeredness 197
self-conficence 48
Self-Examination 96, 101, 103
self-exhaltation 74
Self-Existing, The 44, 186
self-restraining 111
Self-Restraint 70
self-restraint 67, 72, 78, 111
sensation 95
sensory aspects of self 217
servanthood 207
Servanthood, Moving Towards 118
servants 129
Serving God's Creation 118
sex 68, 79, 99
Shabistarī 166
shahīd 89, 166, 232
Shahīd, al- 39, 166
shakūr 87, 150, 152, 153
Shakūr, al- 25, 87, 153
Shaper of Unique Beauty 13, 14, 72, 131
shaykh 122
shepherd 135
Sign (s) 89, 163
Signs of Divine Power 88
Signs of Divine Wisdom 88
Signs of God 144
Signs, Our 22
silver 171
Sincerity 97, 107
slander 88
slayer 76
Slayer, The 43
snake (s) 128, 134, 176, 177
Social Awakening 115, 116
socioethics 227
Solomon 145, 155, 1256, 167, 168, 169, 224
soul 9
Source 92, 112
Source of All Goodness 52, 109, 201, 202
sovereign 95, 99, 124, 141
Sovereign, The 7, 8, 9
sovereignty 121
soverign 228
sperm 37
Spirit 7
Spiritual Poverty 69
Spiritual Power 159
Spiritual Power to Help Others, Using Their 117
spiritual poverty 77, 78
spiritual power 103, 164
Straight Path 79, 128, 134, 141, 145, 202
strength 41
strong 105
Strong, The 40, 41

subduer 100
Subduer, The 15
sublte 145
Submission 69
subtle 102
Subtle, The 17, 23, 103, 146
Sultan 194
sunnah 73, 231
Surah Hūd 93
symbol 218

T
takbīr 13
takbīr al-iḥrām 125
taqwā 74. 150, 201
tattoo 150
tawbah 202
tawwāb 91, 92, 193, 202, 233
Tawwāb, al- 52, 202
Teacher to Others, 118
temperance 67, 68, 78, 111, 140, 142, 186, 197
thankful 87, 150, 152, 153
Thankfulness 81
thankfulness 87, 88, 89, 154
Thankfulness, The Rewarder of 25, 87
theoethics 109, 227
thorns 181
Throne 139
Tradition (s) 8, 58, 67, 71, 80, 83, 84, 88, 142, 160, 163, 164
Tranquillity 69
tranquillity 76
Trust 81
trust 90
trustee 172
Trustee, The 40, 90, 173
trusteeship 172
Trusting in God 117
Trustworthy 174
truth 104, 138, 140, 141
Truth, The 39, 167
Truthfulness 97
truthfulness 104, 105, 230
Turk 123
Turning to God 202

U
'Umar, Caliph 154, 155
ummah 131
unconscious 67
unique 106
unique beauty 131, 132
Unique, The 46
Unity 97
unity 106
unity in multiplicity 46
usefulness 11, 12
uzum 123

V
vainglory 89
vast 103
Vast, The 32
Vigilance 81
vigilant 89, 159, 161
Vigilant, The 31
volition 95

W, X, Y, Z
wadūd 159, 164, 232
Wadūd, al- 34, 89, 153
wahhāb 131, 133, 230
Wahhāb, al- 16, 35, 86, 133, 165
waḥīd 106, 183, 190, 232
Waḥīd, al- 46
wajh 55
wajīd 105, 183, 187
Wajīd, al- 45
wakīl 172, 232
Wakīl, al- 40, 90, 173
wālī (*walī*) 77, 95, 172, 193, 200, 232

Wālī, al- (Walī, al-) 41, 90, 175, 233
wārith 217
Wārith, al- 62, 78, 233
wāsi‘ 103, 232
Wāsi‘, al- 32
water-carrier 222
wave 220
weeds 140
Will of God 106
will power 12, 71, 73, 107, 132
wisdom 39, 48, 95, 96, 144
wise 103, 163
Wise, The 33
witness 89, 166
Witness, The 39
wolf 162
wolves 134
Word of God 134, 144
worldly desires 183
wronging others 127
Zachariah 195
ẓāhir 233
Ẓāhir, al- 50, 108, 199
zeal 84
zealous 84